Autism and Child Psycho

C000137494

Series editor

Johnny L. Matson, Baton Rouge, LA, USA

More information about this series at http://www.springer.com/series/8665

Teresa A. Cardon
Editor

Technology and the Treatment of Children with Autism Spectrum Disorder

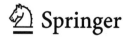 Springer

Editor
Teresa A. Cardon
Utah Valley University
Orem, UT
USA

ISSN 2192-922X   ISSN 2192-9238   (electronic)
Autism and Child Psychopathology Series
ISBN 978-3-319-37175-7   ISBN 978-3-319-20872-5   (eBook)
DOI 10.1007/978-3-319-20872-5

Springer International Publishing AG Switzerland is part of Springer Science+Business Media
(www.springer.com)

First and foremost I would like to dedicate this book to the many families and individuals with autism that have inspired the intensive research and treatments presented on these pages.

I must also take this opportunity to dedicate this book to my sweet Grandma Joy. I know you would have loved the final product! And of course, a shout of appreciation to my own parents, Carol & Jan, who often have more faith in me than I have in myself!

To my children, Rylee and Breelyn, thank you for supporting me as I pursue so many different opportunities. I look forward to returning the favor as you venture, headstrong, into your futures! My heart to you both!

And to Craig, who has found me many a night, typing away into the wee hours of the morning, thank you! Thank you for "getting me" in a way that no one else does. I happily pen this dedication to you knowing that you already understand!

Acknowledgments

I must first thank Dr. Johnny Matson for entrusting me with this exciting project. I must also thank Judy Jones and Michelle Tam for their support in bringing this work to fruition, and a special thanks to Julie Nelson for her meticulous eye and patience with every page.

I am deeply grateful to the many talented researchers, educators, and devoted clinicians who have graciously shared their expertise inside each chapter. I am humbled every day that I get to learn from such talented and dedicated individuals. I am excited that your contributions will benefit so many and personally thank you for your involvement.

Contents

About the Editor

Teresa A. Cardon Ph.D., CCC-SLP, has worked with individuals on the autism spectrum for more than 20 years. Dr. Cardon completed her doctoral training in Speech and Hearing Science with an autism emphasis and is currently the Director of Autism Studies at Utah Valley University. Dr. Cardon continues to publish her research on autism in peer-reviewed journals and presents at conferences both nationally and internationally. Dr. Cardon's first line of research focuses on video modeling with young children with autism. Her second line of research focuses on fictional narratives with character's who have an ASD. She is the author of three books that offer intervention support for individuals on the autism spectrum: *Top Ten Tips* (2008), *Initiations and Interactions* (2006), and *Let's Talk Emotions* (2004).

Contributors

Laura Linnell Anderson University of Utah, Salt Lake City, UT, USA

Kevin M. Ayres The University of Georgia, Athens, GA, USA

Teresa A. Cardon Utah Valley University, Orem, UT, USA

Amy Bixler Coffin Ohio Center for Autism and Low Incidence, Columbus, OH, USA

Marissa Lynn Diener University of Utah, Salt Lake City, UT, USA

Karen H. Douglas Illinois State University, Normal, IL, USA

Terisa P. Gabrielsen Brigham Young University, Provo, UT, USA

Phyllis Jones University of South Florida, Tampa, FL, USA

Kristi A. Jordan Indiana Resource Center for Autism, Indiana University, Bloomington, IN, USA

Ryan O. Kellems Brigham Young University, Provo, UT, USA

Justin D. Lane The University of Kentucky, Lexington, KY, USA

Kristie Brown Lofland Indiana Resource Center for Autism, Indiana University, Bloomington, IN, USA

Georgina T.F. Lynch Washington State University, Spokane, WA, USA

Riley's Mom Utah Autism Academy, Midvale, UT, USA

Brenda Smith Myles Ohio Center for Autism and Low Incidence, Columbus, OH, USA

Tricia Nelson Utah Autism Academy, Midvale, UT, USA

Jan Rogers Ohio Center for Autism and Low Incidence, Columbus, OH, USA

Collin Shepley Oconee County Schools, Watkinsville, GA, USA

Sally B. Shepley The University of Georgia, Athens, GA, USA

Jodie Simon A Division of Jigsaw Learning, LLC, Teachtown, Woburn, MA, USA

Wendy Szakacs Ohio Center for Autism and Low Incidence, Columbus, OH, USA

Catherine Wilcox University of South Florida, Tampa, FL, USA

Caroline Williams Brigham Young University, Provo, UT, USA

Cheryl A. Wright University of Utah, Salt Lake City, UT, USA

Scott D. Wright University of Utah, Salt Lake City, UT, USA

Chapter 1
An Introduction

Teresa A. Cardon

The prevalence rates of autism spectrum disorder (ASD) have increased rapidly over the past 20 years with 1 in 68 children currently being diagnosed (CDC 2014). As more and more children have been diagnosed with the disorder, the search to find a cause has intensified and researchers have continued to uncover more and more indicators (e.g., Gardener et al. 2011; Rosenberg et al. 2009; National Autism Center 2009). Due to this increase, the search for appropriate and effective interventions has become a priority (e.g., Ayres and Langone 2005; Koegel and Koegel 2006). Interestingly, as the autism rates have been escalating, a surge in technology has been taking place.

Twenty years ago, there were no smartphones or tablet computers and laptops were not as everyday as were desktop computers. Access to the Internet was not commonplace, and wireless components were few and far between. Fast-forward to 2014, and it is not uncommon for single households to own multiple devices, and smartphone use has surpassed that of personal computers (O'Toole 2014). But how has this surge in technology affected the intervention aspects of people impacted by ASD?

Historically, technology has been used to support individuals diagnosed with ASD in a variety of ways. For example, speech output devices have provided augmented communication for individuals who were unable to verbally express themselves (Beukelman and Mirenda 1992). Computers have acted as educational aids to assist children with reading, writing, and instruction (e.g., Heimann et al. 1995; Higgins and Boone 1996). And, video cameras have been used since the turn of the century to record and provide video models of important skills that children with autism needed to learn (Charlop-Chirsty et al. 2000).

With the influx of technology, particularly with regard to smartphones, tablets, and wireless capabilities, the use of technology to support intervention for individuals with autism has shifted. The purpose of this book is to provide insight into how technology has advanced and to specifically address practical ways that the reader can use technology, both hardware and software, with the individuals they

T.A. Cardon (✉)
Utah Valley University, Orem, UT, USA
e-mail: Teresa.cardon@uvu.edu

© Springer International Publishing Switzerland 2016
T.A. Cardon (ed.), *Technology and the Treatment of Children with Autism Spectrum Disorder*, Autism and Child Psychopathology Series,
DOI 10.1007/978-3-319-20872-5_1

serve. The most up-to-date research will be presented to help readers identify best practice approaches. Our goal is to present new ideas and strategies that will improve the lives of individuals with autism through the use of technology.

References

Ayres, K. M., & Langone, J. (2005). Intervention and instruction with video for students with autism: A review of the literature. *Education and Training in Developmental Disabilities, 40* (2), 183–196.

Beukelman, D., & Mirenda, P. (1992). *Augmentative and alternative communication: Management of severe communication disorders in children and adults*. Baltimore: Paul H. Brookes.

Center for Disease Control. (CDC; 2014). Data and statistics—autism spectrum disorders—risks and characteristics. Retrieved July 11, 2014 from http://www.cdc.gov/ncbddd/autism/data.html.

Charlop-Christy, M. H., Le, L., & Freeman, K. (2000). A comparison of video modeling with in vivo modeling for teaching children with autism. *Journal of Autism and Developmental Disorders, 30*, 537–552.

Gardener, H., Spiegelman, D., & Buka, S. L. (2011). Perinatal and neonatal risk factors for autism: A comprehensive meta-analysis. *Pediatrics, 128*(2), 344–355.

Heimann, M., Nelson, K. E., Tjus, T., & Gillberg, C. (1995). Increasing reading and communication skills in children with autism through an interactive multimedia computer program. *Journal of Autism and Developmental Disorders, 25*(5), 459–480.

Higgins, K., & Boone, R. (1996). Creating individualized computer-assisted instruction for students with autism using multimedia authoring software. *Focus on Autism and Other Developmental Disabilities, 11*(2), 69–78.

Koegel, R., & Koegel, L. (2006). *Pivotal Response Treatments for Autism* (pp. 141–159). Baltimore, MD: Paul H. Brookes Publishing Co.

National Autism Center. (2009). *National Standards Report: The national standards project—addressing the need for evidence-based practice guidelines for autism spectrum disorders*.

O'Toole, J. (2014). *Mobile apps overtake PC Internet usage in U.S.* Retrieved on July 11, 2014 from http://money.cnn.com/2014/02/28/technology/mobile/mobile-apps-internet/.

Rosenberg, R. E., Law, J. K., Yenokyan, G., McGready, J., Kaufmann, W. E., & Law, P. A. (2009). Characteristics and concordance of autism spectrum disorders among 277 twin pairs. *Archives of Pediatric and Adolescent Medicine, 163*(10), 907–914.

Chapter 2
AAC for Individuals with Autism Spectrum Disorder: Assessment and Establishing Treatment Goals

Georgina T.F. Lynch

Introduction

An area of great interest to clinicians, holding promise with current technology to support the individual with autism spectrum disorder (ASD), is that of augmentative and alternative communication (AAC) as part of a comprehensive intensive treatment approach to address communication needs. Although great strides have been made in the area of technology to support the use of AAC with individuals with communication disorders, the use of AAC with the ASD population is often the least understood by the practicing clinician in terms of efficacy and how to establish a foundation for developing an effective language and communication system that sustains over time. Due to the many behavioral challenges found with ASD, basic pre-linguistic behaviors necessary to benefit from AAC are often overlooked in the early stages of assessment and treatment, and the advanced AAC systems put into place frequently become abandoned due to the lack of engagement with the technology on the part of the individual with ASD, resulting in minimal improvements in functional communication. Despite the challenges that exist when introducing AAC to children or adults with ASD, establishing a foundation for where to begin, promoting successful engagement with the device as a communication tool, and developing a true language system for the child are all attainable goals if comprehensive evaluation of behavior and language are completed prior to the introduction of any AAC device. The remainder of this chapter will focus on evaluation and development of language and communication skills necessary to support the introduction of AAC, emphasizing the introduction of technology to young children with a diagnosis of ASD, although a similar approach can be taken with older adolescents and young adults as well. Given what is known about the plasticity of the brain early in development (Dawson 2008; Helt et al. 2008), and given current

G.T.F. Lynch (✉)
Washington State University, Spokane, WA, USA
e-mail: georgina.lynch@wsu.edu

© Springer International Publishing Switzerland 2016
T.A. Cardon (ed.), *Technology and the Treatment of Children with Autism Spectrum Disorder*, Autism and Child Psychopathology Series,
DOI 10.1007/978-3-319-20872-5_2

3

outcome data related to intensive early intervention with a focus on the functional analysis of behavior and language development (Dawson et al. 2010; National Autism Center 2015), the information presented hereafter related to assessment and establishing treatment goals will be provided using the lens of early intervention to support optimal response to the introduction of AAC. The reader must bear in mind that principles for applying the use of AAC to individuals with autism do not change due to an individual's age, but are best applied early on in development, so as to capitalize on the development of a true language system by targeting key characteristics of behavior and communication that result from neurologic deficits known to be present in the ASD brain. Such deficits may include difficulty with motor planning and coordination of oral musculature to produce oral speech, difficulty with auditory comprehension of language, slow processing of synaptic activity between brain regions resulting in delayed responding or complete lack of response, and difficulty with inhibition of impulsive behavior due to differences in amygdala response and frontal lobe activity (Amaral et al. 2008). It is important to consider these behaviors in the context of implementing AAC in order to increase the response to intervention by merging behavioral intervention with cognitive and language intervention that supports increasing synaptic pathways that facilitate expressive language and potentially, verbal speech production.

Given the heterogeneity of the ASD presenting phenotype, this chapter will examine current technology regarding options available for low-level basic communication needs and explore high-tech options available to address early literacy and social/pragmatic needs for individuals diagnosed with ASD with less impacted language skills, but for whom social pragmatic deficits pose difficulty in more advanced use and understanding of abstract language and socially appropriate behaviors. Recent changes to the Diagnostic and Statistical Manual of Mental Disorders, Fifth Edition-DSM-5 (American Psychiatric Association 2013), identify individuals with ASD in terms of the level of support needed in an attempt to subtype varying degrees of severity of ASD. As the individual with ASD develops skills, the diagnosis may remain, but the level of support may change over time. An interpretation of "Level of Support" as described under the Autism diagnostic criteria in the DSM-5 may be interpreted by what supports may be needed in the form of physical assistance, medications, and potential AAC, among other interventions. Just as the range of behaviors and needs are varied with the diagnosis of ASD, so are the AAC options to support language and communication, regardless of level of severity on the spectrum.

AAC: Defining AAC: Implications for the Application of AAC to the ASD Population

To fully understand the various types of AAC available and what type of technology may best support the individual with autism, background knowledge about types of AAC and frequently used terminology is helpful in determining the options that may be available, and those options most likely to offer success in terms of their use with ASD. The American Speech-Language Hearing Association (2014) defines AAC as including "…all forms of communication (other than oral speech) that are used to express thoughts, needs, wants, and ideas. We all use AAC when we make facial expressions or gestures, use symbols or pictures, or write." Implied within this definition is the use of conventional forms of communication and abstract language, which poses the greatest challenge to the child with ASD. Given the complexity of the needs and behavioral challenges, when considering the use of AAC with the autism population, the process for assessment should include an inter-professional team with specialized knowledge and skills related to AAC. To offer full potential for successful introduction to AAC technology, in addition to experience with AAC, each member of the team should also hold some degree of expertise in treating individuals with autism, as the unique nature of the associated behaviors requires an understanding of how to address challenging behavior, typical patterns of difficulty related to learning verbal speech and language, and how to incorporate AAC intervention within the broader behavioral program that addresses other developmental domains such as adaptive skills, cognitive skills, and social interaction and play. Effective treatment for speech and language intervention when paired with AAC requires ongoing continuing education and clinical training in terms of knowledge and application of skills that include the use of evidence-based practices (American Speech-Language Hearing Association 2004). Typically, an AAC team serving individuals with ASD includes the clinical psychologist or school-psychologist, the speech-language pathologist, the certified behavior analyst, the occupational therapist, the parent or caregiver, and other special education educators and personnel interacting daily with the child. The speech-language pathologist often will guide development of the treatment goals, given the expertise in the area of language development. Collaboration and consultation among team members is essential to achieve goals related to communication. The complexity of the AAC intervention program is as unique and varied as the individuals identified with ASD and should adapt and change as the individual's needs and skills change. Therefore, collaboration and ongoing dynamic assessment throughout the AAC intervention program is necessary. A foundation of understanding among team members regarding AAC options, AAC terminology, and the current research related to AAC and autism is helpful as teams embark on this aspect of the individual's treatment program.

Types of AAC: Unaided and Aided

There are two primary forms of AAC used with individuals with communication disorders: *unaided and aided AAC*. Whereas aided AAC requires the use of adaptive equipment and tools, unaided AAC does not require additional equipment to support the alternative communication use in the absence of verbal speech. The individual uses his or her body to convey messages, ideas, and needs, and this form of AAC may include sign and gestures. The most commonly used form of unaided alternative communication includes the use of sign language. Although universally accepted as an effective communication tool for the deaf population with an established language system, the use of sign language tends to be less effective in building language for individuals with ASD due to inherent challenges with imitation, difficulty with initiation of communication, and the lack of understanding of sign by the communication partners encountered throughout one's day (Frost and Bondy 2002; National Autism Center 2015). Quite often in cases of ASD, the speech-language pathologist may introduce AAC by supplementing it with the use of simple signs to convey messages to the individual paired with behavioral intervention, such as presenting the signs for "Stop," "More," "Help," and "All done." However, it is important to note that the use of these functional signs would mostly be considered unaided AAC in the form of *gesture, as opposed to sign language*, because these signs are often taught as a way of providing visual support for communication attempts and comprehension of early language forms. The signs are not used to build an expressive language system. Given that the visual modality is often an area of strength for the child with ASD, these simple gestures may be used with repetition when paired with verbal reinforcement to help the child with ASD begin to associate the sound of words with meaning. Therefore, simple signs may be used to supplement initial stages of teaching related to imitation and understanding of abstract language concepts. The emphasis on the gestural aspect of these signs, paired with behavioral reinforcement and verbal speech models are the key components supporting those very early stages of communicative interactions for the individual with ASD and do not support the development of a long-term signing vocabulary or sign language system. The use of unaided AAC in the form of sign language is of little support to the individual with ASD because children with ASD do not follow a typical trajectory for language and cognitive development, which relies heavily on established pre-linguistic behaviors such as imitation, pointing, joint attention, initiating communication with caregivers, and understanding cause and effect (Kaderavek 2011). These challenges related to the use of pre-linguistic behaviors are often accompanied by extreme difficulty expressing wants and needs, resulting in the use of unconventional forms of communication to get needs met, such as screaming, lying on the floor, hitting others, or grabbing objects. Since the child with ASD typically may not possess imitation skills, gestural skills, or a functional emerging language system in the absence of verbal speech, as opposed to infants and toddlers with delayed expressive language, or as with children who are deaf or hard of hearing, when an adult signs to the child with ASD, there is little generalization toward language use.

The most effective form of AAC for children with ASD is the use of aided AAC, relying on visual support in the form of objects, pictures, and video. Based on a review of 389 studies regarding treatment efficacy, the National Standards Report (National Autism Center 2015), considered among ASD research scientists and specialists to be the guiding document for the use of evidence-based practices, identified the use of AAC as an "emerging" treatment, considered to hold positive outcomes for children of all ages and levels of severity on the spectrum. Further research regarding specific components that support the effectiveness of AAC intervention with the ASD population is still needed to fully understand the critical elements of its use with language intervention impacting long-term outcomes. The current body of the research literature related to AAC and autism is limited in its generalization due to the small samples sizes and the heterogeneity of the samples. However, when paired with intensive interventions utilizing principles of applied behavior analysis, results have been replicated indicating AAC as an intervention holding promise in promoting an increase in expressive language and functional communication (Dawson et al. 2010; National Autism Center 2015).

It is widely understood by clinicians who work with individuals with ASD that often there is a need to provide visual support to improve the child's response to intervention, and that most effective intervention programs include some form of explicit visual teaching (Mesibov et al. 2004; National Research Council 2001; Dawson and Osterling 1997). However, of recent interest in the literature, is what individuals with ASD pay attention to in terms of visual processing, as a way of understanding how best to use AAC. The use of eye-tracking technology is improving our understanding of this aspect of behavior that has a direct impact on outcomes related to AAC intervention (Gillespie-Smith and Fletcher-Watson 2014). In a study by Hernandez et al. (2009), significant differences in visual attending and eye gaze were found in individuals with ASD when compared to controls, with the ASD group demonstrating a lack of visual attention to faces in comparison with objects, reduced fixation toward the eyes, and an increase in observation toward the mouth when viewing human faces. These findings have been replicated (Pelphrey et al. 2002; Riby and Hancock 2009) and offer support for translating this research into the use of AAC, given the heavy reliance on the visual system to benefit from this technology. As children with ASD are acquiring language, often there exists sensory overload in terms of noise, touch, and scent, which impact their ability to process incoming verbal information. fMRI research in the area of audio–visual integration in the ASD brain indicates difficulty with unimodal stimuli, but an increase in cortical activation and connection when individuals with ASD are trained to listen and watch at the same time, thus providing the basis for using visual support in teaching language-based concepts and verbal speech (Williams et al. 2004). Capitalizing on the use of visual support with aided AAC helps the individual with autism increase focus and attention to visual stimuli that may be paired with verbal input to increase the association between abstract language and verbal speech. The additional benefit of aided AAC is that visual stimuli can be adapted to meet the needs of the individual in terms of presentation, such as the use of black and white symbols, line drawings, photos, and even objects if needed.

Aided AAC is frequently the first line of intervention early on as speech-language pathologists' work with children with ASD because of its emphasis on visual support. Whereas it is necessary to determine where to start with AAC and where to go with it in terms of language development, as AAC is implemented with the child with autism, verbal speech may begin to emerge when intervention is paired with some form of visual support. Mirenda et al. (2013) analyzed treatment outcomes for a cohort of 191 Canadian children diagnosed with ASD who had received intensive early intervention and AAC support, which yielded interesting results regarding the attainment of verbal speech by six years of age. 38.2 % of the children had a baseline vocabulary of 5 words or fewer at the time of initial diagnosis and represented only 10.5 % of children remaining in need of AAC at six years of age. 31.4 % of the children had single words and no phrases and comprised 14.1 % of the low-verbal group at six years of age. These changes represented a collective reduction from 69.4 to 24.6 % of children in need of AAC support, indicating a trend toward acquisition of verbal speech when intensive early intervention had been provided, commensurate with current findings related to early intervention treatment outcomes for programs emphasizing language and behavioral intervention (Dawson et al. 2010). Thus, the AAC may serve as an initial catalyst to teach the abstract language and may be faded out in the intervention process as verbal speech is acquired and an emerging language system is developed. In other cases, the AAC will become a lifelong need, specifically when there is comorbid apraxia of speech or other difficulty with motor planning for speech production, and cognitive deficits. In the former case, consideration for AAC use as an advanced language system including the development of literacy will need to be addressed early in the establishment of treatment goals.

Introduction of AAC: Transitioning from Low- to High-Tech AAC Options

Most clinicians working with individuals with ASD can identify a family or two for whom they recall the parent holding the perception that the promise of an iPAD© might be the "window to their child's voice" and the hope of "opening the door for communication." Often it may have been perceived that if only they had this high-tech device, everything else would fall into place on its own. Unfortunately, whether it is an iPAD©, a Vanguard©, or a GoTalk20©, if assessment is not thorough relative to the pre-linguistic behaviors and unconventional forms of communication currently observed, the outcomes for functional communication and/or verbal speech based on the use of these advanced or high-tech options may be limited. When a thorough, comprehensive evaluation regarding essential pre-linguistic skills is completed, the AAC technology truly does open a whole new world to the child. As assessment is discussed, the reader will have a more thorough understanding of decision-making relative to the use of high-tech AAC options, well beyond knowledge of brands or commonly recognized devices. It is important to establish some preliminary observations relative to the use of AAC in order to establish treatment goals and to determine the capabilities of the child to grow with a device, as well as to match the capabilities of the device over the long term to support the child's needs.

Given this path of dynamic assessment as a process toward developing functional AAC use, often it is best to initially consider some low-tech options as a way of measuring the potential for success, in order to put into place some immediate visual support to address behavior and to begin the early intensive teaching process. Low-tech options include the use of picture boards, "Big Mac" buttons that initiate a question or comment, and the use of the Picture Exchange Communication System (PECS, Frost and Bondy 2002). All of these systems are effective for establishing some initial communication and for completing informal observations during evaluation of pre-linguistic communication skills such as demonstration of cause and effect, imitation, joint attention, visual discrimination, and initiations. Low-tech options fail children with ASD when a team has recommended its use and then did not follow through to advance the child beyond these simple forms of communication fairly early on in the treatment program. A plateau will occur and the child will not use the emerging language skills if the AAC does not advance and adapt. When used as part of the initial assessment process and during the early stages of intervention to teach basic skills, low-tech options can be quite productive to establish basic communicative behaviors without the distraction of high-tech devices that often create more intrigue for the child in terms of visual display, noise, and light, resulting in counterproductive behaviors. Although highly motivating to the child with ASD in terms of engagement with these high-tech devices, when introduced too early without establishing the aforementioned basic communicative behaviors, the use of AAC sometimes becomes a behavioral intervention challenge more than a language system intervention. Thus, it behooves the conscientious clinician to begin with low-tech AAC in order to establish baseline behaviors related to functional communication, and then gradually transition to high-tech options as these skills emerge. This approach often does not take much time at all and can be accomplished over a series of 8–10 sessions or a few weeks, if paired with intensive behavioral support.

Before examining the assessment process in more detail, in order to make these difficult decisions regarding device choice, one must have an understanding of the types of technology options available on various devices. Given how much has changed over the past decade or so in terms of the technology, a number of speech-language pathologists and behavior interventionists have chosen to specialize in the area of AAC in order to stay abreast of current technology. The twenty-first century has seen exponential growth in technology options available for AAC ranging from traditional dedicated speech generating devices to the recent cost effective application options available on most operating system platforms which are easily accessible to the general public. Given this technological world we now live in, it is quite common for typically developing children and adolescents in public school settings to be familiar with AAC devices and see their peers using these devices, in comparison with the use of AAC prior to 2000. Therefore, the use of AAC devices within the common population is increasing and widely accepted among society, much like the use of sign language. Just as with other forms of technology, the development of innovative AAC technology options for individuals with communication needs has emerged as an area of economic growth, while also improving quality of life and independence for people with a variety of communication disorders.

Types of High-Tech AAC Options

The following types of options are available on most high-tech devices and are commonly used terms to describe the capability of AAC systems: *fixed display, dynamic display, visual scene display (VSD), and speech generating device (SGD)*. In a fixed display option, symbols and messages remain static on the screen after a symbol is selected, therefore nothing changes and images are always present in the same position, regardless of whether a symbol is chosen or not. The use of a fixed display is helpful early in the process of teaching AAC use, especially with children with ASD, because it offers preliminary practice with cause and effect and visual discrimination. The fixed display allows for ease of self-correction for mis-hits, and is fairly easy to use because there are limited navigation challenges, as there are with devices that use dynamic displays. In addition, predictability and routine are intricately connected to the use of the fixed display, as all symbols are always found in exactly the same place; the predictability can be very helpful for the individual with ASD struggling with emotional regulation, because less cognitive demand is placed on expressing wants and needs in the moment when trying to communicate.

By contrast, the dynamic display option offers a great amount of flexibility in terms of access to vocabulary and conceptualization of the vocabulary and tends to offer a more advanced language system feature for developing stronger semantic skills and syntax variability, both skills necessary for developing advanced language and literacy. A dynamic display option changes the screen display once a symbol is selected. For example, by selecting a symbol that looks like an apple, the screen may then open to a new screen with a variety of food options. Therefore, the symbol for apple becomes representative for the category of "foods." One can see how quickly the cognitive demands change from the fixed display option to the dynamic display option. The person using AAC with the dynamic display option and the example above now must have an understanding of categories, multiple steps related to cause and effect, and reasoning skills to begin to put ideas together, in comparison with the more simplistic process of selecting a picture that holds a one-to-one correspondence with the object or concept, as with the fixed display option. Dynamic displays offer much more in terms of options for the device to evolve as the child's language development evolves, and therefore they are often used with children for whom there is higher receptive language ability and a need for more complex language use.

Whereas both the fixed display and dynamic display options focus on the use of symbol cells (boxes on the screen with a symbol embedded within each box), which are selected to communicate, VSD options embed pictures of desired objects, needs, and ideas, within visual context. The message is conveyed by selecting an image from a visual scene depicting a picture that includes the communication "symbol" or image, within a scene holding some relevant meaning or context for its use. For example, instead of selecting an icon for "food" such as an apple icon, a bowl of fruit on the table in a picture scene of a kitchen becomes the symbol to select communication messages about food, specifically fruits and vegetables. Emerging studies in the area of autism research have focused on the use of VSDs and visual processing (Wilkinson et al. 2012). Of critical importance to access the available AAC technology options is the consideration of eye-tracking data cited in studies of ASD to measure attention to the visual stimuli and selection of symbols for communication. In a study analyzing gaze fixation, Wilkinson and Light (2014) found that school-age children with ASD paid visual attention to faces of people embedded within picture scenes, even in the presence of other distracting objects, supporting the use of VSDs with the ASD population. Given the characteristic challenges with eye contact, and a preference of individuals with autism to attend to objects more than faces (Hadjikhani et al. 2004), the focus on objects within an environment that are contextually rich and include "hot spots," or specific areas of the picture, lends itself very well to supporting the individual with ASD in acquiring language. VSDs tend to be more concrete than isolated symbolic icons and provide a context for using and understanding the language associated with the vocabulary incorporated into the scene (Beukelman and Mirenda 2013). The use of VSDs offers a new format for using AAC with the ASD population and addresses some of the challenges related to the generalization of communication skills to other contexts, since the vocabulary is used within the specific context or setting it would be anticipated to most often be needed.

Regardless of whether or not a fixed display, dynamic display, or VSD option is selected, all of these options can be found in a SGD. The SGD provides voice output as the child selects the picture or symbol to communicate. SGDs provide a verbal model for the individual, reinforcing the use of the word with the symbol as the child uses the SGD to communicate wants and needs. In addition, because the device "speaks" for the child, there is no need for the communication partner to understand a different language system, and the child begins to be reinforced for communication attempts that follow the typical grammatical pattern for using oral language. SGDs are also available in the form of applications on mobile and tablet devices and are therefore cost-effective options for meeting basic communication needs out in the community and in the home with familiar communication partners. In the case of children with ASD who may already possess some verbal ability, the use of the SGD may promote an increase in social initiations and fewer communication breakdowns with unfamiliar communication partners and is emerging in the research as a preferred mode of communication among young children with autism (van der Meer et al. 2012). Furthermore, it is imperative that clinicians explain the relationship between verbal language development and the use of AAC to families when considering AAC as part of their child's intervention program. Sometimes parents may be concerned that the use of PECS or SGDs may hinder their child's oral language development. However, the current empirical literature in the area of ASD and AAC use indicates that the use of AAC does not inhibit the development of verbal speech and may, in fact, promote acquisition of verbal speech, if intervention is provided at an intensive rate early in development (Mirenda 2013). Parents can be reassured that the AAC may be used to provide a tool to the child for basic communication and to teach language, and if the child begins to demonstrate verbal ability, the AAC supplements the use of verbal speech and may serve to foster more advanced verbal language development.

The distinction in AAC as a *tool for communication as opposed to the language system for communication* is essential to the understanding of the strengths and limitations of AAC with the ASD population. The AAC alone does not teach the child language nor does its use suddenly make the non-verbal child verbal and socially engaging. The AAC is the scaffold by which the speech-language pathologist and other specialists support communication to meet daily needs and to help the child benefit from intervention targeting more advanced language use. AAC use focused on basic communication in the absence of explicit, structured language intervention to promote a more sophisticated language system, results in little positive long-term outcomes related to cognitive and academic skills, often resulting in a plateau in terms of progress. Much like tapping into the full range of potential of a complex computer system, without basic knowledge of the underlying language needed to use the AAC, the user does not fully realize its optimal use. If we do not build the child's language system taking a developmental approach, there will be gaps in the child's communicative competence and an unsteady foundation upon which the AAC is being used. It is essential that the technology being used match the child's emerging developmental language level.

Primary Areas to Address When Assessing for AAC and Education for the Family

The primary goal of an evaluation for AAC with a child diagnosed with autism should be to fully assess the pre-linguistic behaviors needed to benefit from learning and those skills needed to understand the use of the AAC as a communication tool. The most frequently identified goal for the family of a child with autism is the desire to communicate with their child and understand what the child wants. The impact of the autism diagnosis on the family is unlike that of any other childhood communication disorder, and the use of AAC holds promise for those families. When measuring cortisol levels, Mailick Seltzer et al. (2009) found that the stress level in mothers of adolescents with ASD was comparable to that of combat veterans presenting with symptoms of post-traumatic stress disorder. The constant management of safety needs and intense behaviors due to the lack of communication ability also takes its toll on families. Hartley et al. (2010) examined the divorce rate among parents of children with ASD and found that divorce rate was slightly higher than typical families, falling at 23.5 % regardless of the age of the child, in comparison with a representative sample of parents without a child with ASD, at 13.8 %. There is no doubt the impact of ASD among the general population has risen to a level of public health concern in the USA, as well as across the globe (Centers for Disease Control and Prevention 2014; World Health Organization 2013), with parents looking for that silver bullet to make their child's life better and to bring a "voice" to their child who can only express himself/herself through unconventional means of communication. Implementation of AAC should be carefully explained to families in terms of its potential to resolve communication challenges, but it should also be emphasized that there will still be the need for intensive language and behavioral intervention to make its use successful.

There is often urgency around providing some form of communication for the individual to express wants and needs, due to the severity of behaviors and due to the intense desire of parents to communicate with their child. Under these circumstances, parents and providers alike sometimes believe if only the child had the means to communicate, everything would be different. In this kind of scenario, often the use of AAC is viewed by families as the means by which the child's challenges will be solved and the bridge to communication will be established. When implementation of AAC is done well, this may very well be the case; when done out of urgency, without proper consideration of all aspects of the child's developmental areas, and when monitored by clinicians not familiar with the complexities of the development of linguistic competence, often parents' hopes of communication and building a relationship with the child may be lost. It is not uncommon for specialists in the area of behavior intervention to propose the use of AAC or even recommend a particular device for the child with autism, without possessing the knowledge and skills related to the complexities of language development. This approach can be problematic when AAC recommendations are given from a behavioral standpoint related to functional communication, as opposed to providing recommendations from a broader developmental standpoint that includes analysis of behavior, adaptive skills, and specific cognitive skills related to the development of language. In order to fully realize the optimal benefit of AAC technology, fundamental pre-linguistic skills and behaviors must be in place to support use of the AAC and careful assessment of these skills will support more successful use of AAC for improving communication and developing language skills.

Prior to learning oral language, typically developing children demonstrate specific skills that are conducive to further developing communicative competence and subsequent oral language which include skills related to object permanence, cause and effect, joint attention, and imitation (Piaget 1953; Kaderavek 2011). Figure 2.1 illustrates a conceptual framework for considering key elements in the evaluation process that includes assessment of fundamental skills and analysis of motivation to use AAC, which should be considered at the initial stages of assessment as part of a comprehensive evaluation for the individual with autism. In addition to cognitive skills, other fundamental skills such as joint attention, eye gaze, engagement with tasks, and visual discrimination are essential to establish a foundation for determining a baseline upon which to begin to build the AAC relative to the child's developmental level.

Thorough assessment of cognitive ability and pre-linguistic behaviors must be addressed as part of comprehensive assessment, which may also include analysis of

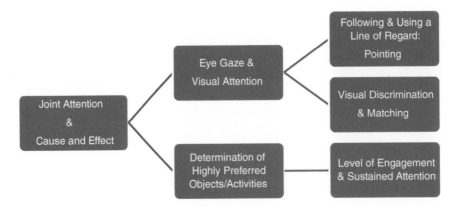

Fig. 2.1 Fundamental cognitive and behavioral skills to assess during the initial stages of comprehensive AAC evaluation for individuals with ASD

factors related to behavioral reinforcement and motivation. The AAC needs of the individual with ASD are unique when compared to other users of AAC, due to the hallmark deficits in social reciprocity and social communication from a pre-linguistic standpoint. Whereas non-verbal children with other communication disorders such as cerebral palsy, childhood apraxia of speech, and childhood deafness will rejoice in the opportunity to communicate and be "heard," the child with autism does not see an AAC tool in the same way. Therefore, basic social interaction and non-verbal expressive language skills must be taught first, which is why assessment of fundamental skills early in the process of AAC evaluation is necessary.

In addition to observation and analysis of fundamental communicative skills and behaviors, a forced-choice preference assessment (Fischer 1992) should also be given, to assess the level of reinforcement particular objects or activities may have, so as to offer an initial repertoire of items and activities that may motivate the child to use the AAC. In a forced-choice preference, assessment pairs of objects are presented randomly and the object the child touches first is recorded each time, which results in a percentage of preference of objects relative to others. The power of the reinforcement for each item is also deduced through this process, as the child may select a particular object 100 % of the time, while selecting another preferred object at 75 % of the time, and a "non-preferred" object 0 % of the time. Adding this component to the assessment process is valuable to the clinician posed with the challenge of finding reinforcing items and activities for which the child will communicate. Although parents and familiar caregivers may offer suggestions about preferred items, often there may be a "satiation effect," in which the items have been used too often in attempts to reduce negative behavior, and therefore, the use of these items as reinforcers, especially to teach new skills, has limited power in terms of increasing motivation.

The Evaluation Process and Tools for Assessment

Given the heterogeneity of the ASD population, what is the best approach to take in order to assess pre-linguistic skills? Typically, there are a number of standardized language tests, social/adaptive scales, and cognitive tools administered which may confirm a diagnosis of ASD, but these tools provide little valuable information relative to the development of specific language goals and where to begin the treatment process relative to the use of AAC. Most children diagnosed with autism have typically been evaluated using tools such as the Autism Diagnostic Observation Schedule, Second Edition (ADOS-2; Lord et al. 2001), considered the gold standard for sensitivity and specificity for the Autism diagnosis. The Autism Diagnostic Interview-Revised (ADI-R; Le Couteur et al. 2003) may also have been given, providing some picture into the history of the child's development across key developmental domains and specific behaviors, providing useful information relative to acquisition of skills and any regression in skills. The Childhood Autism Rating Scale (CARS; Schopler and Van Bourgondien 2010) is also a typical screening tool used early in the diagnostic process that provides some information related to communication partners and style of communication in terms of gesture and verbal speech. These tools are all essential to diagnose autism and differentiate the disorder from other developmental delays; however, a useful tool to the speech-language pathologist for measuring communicative behaviors in the non-verbal child with ASD is the Communication Matrix© (Rowland 2004). This criterion-referenced tool breaks down very early communication skills ranging from pre-linguistic to abstract language use in four domains identified as the primary reasons for communicating: social interaction, obtain things, refuse things, and seek and share information. This tool breaks down communication into seven stages of language development, which begin at unconventional levels of communication in the absence of symbolic language, building in complexity from pre-linguistic behaviors to abstract language use, including verbal speech. The seven stages of communication measured on the Communication Matrix are outlined in Table 2.1. These behaviors should be observed in more than one setting over multiple observations, with more than one communication partner, in order to identify the most commonly used forms of communication.

Determining these baselines of communication ability allows the speech-language pathologist, together with the family and other team members, to determine stages at which to begin the use of AAC and to establish a path by which the communication system will develop relative to the individual's use of existing pre-linguistic behaviors. Instead of looking primarily at communicative contexts and partners throughout the individuals daily routines, as most other tools for AAC assessment do, this analysis focuses on prerequisite skills needed to communicate with those partners in varying contexts, resulting in treatment goals that facilitate the incorporation of the AAC tool with the use of evidence-based intervention practices such as Pivotal Response Training (PRT; Koegel and Koegel 2006), Early Start Denver Model (ESDM; Rogers and Dawson 2009), or the Social Communication Emotional

Table 2.1 Summary of seven stages of communication matrix© and observable behaviors

Stage	Form	Symbolic level	Function	Behaviors	PECS phase
I	Pre-intentional behavior	Pre-symbolic without intent	Expresses discomfort, pain, hunger	Vocalizations; facial expressions	
II	Intentional behavior	Pre-symbolic with intent	Expresses interest, pain, hunger, desire to seek out	Vocalizations; eye gaze; facial expressions	
III	Unconventional communication	Pre-symbolic behaviors used to intentionally communicate and considered unconventional because socially unacceptable	Uses behaviors to get needs met; demonstrates an increase in these behaviors when reinforced	Crying; screaming; body movements such as: kicking, hitting, and tugging on others to get needs met	Phases 1 and 2
IV	Conventional communication	Conventional means are used to communicate	Uses communicative initiations and hands and body for interaction	Gesture; nodding or shaking head; looking from object to person; pointing	
V	Concrete symbols	Symbol is physically similar to what is represented: toy teacup for "cup" or "drink"	Initiates communication and one-to-one correspondence with photographs/objects	Pictures, objects given to others to express wants, needs, and ideas	Phase 3
VI	Abstract symbols	Symbolic: may not physically look like the object or idea it represents; e.g., stop sign for "stop"/"all done"	Symbols used one at a time to express ideas	Written words, signs, braille, line drawings	Phase 3
VII[a]	Language	Grammatical rules followed representing abstract concepts	Used in two or three symbol combinations	"I want juice"; "Truck go!"; may be verbal or non-verbal	Levels 4, 5, and 6

Adapted from: Rowland (2004)

[a]Transition to AAC most optimal at communication stage VII and Phase 4 of PECS

Regulation Transactional (SCERTS; Prizant et al. 2006) model to teach the necessary pre-linguistic skills. As previously mentioned, the AAC is the tool, and an evidence-based language intervention will need to be paired with it to yield positive outcomes related to its use. The assessment process within the initial stages of evaluation provides a foundation upon which to establish treatment goals for determining social interaction using pre-linguistic behaviors that promote effective use of the AAC for conventional use of communication and advancement toward more sophisticated development of language. Although the Communication Matrix© is a measure that explicitly describes levels of communication and language, meant to pinpoint where to begin AAC treatment goals, the comprehensive AAC evaluation should also include other measures of adaptive and cognitive tools as well. The reader is referred to Beukelman and Mirenda (2013) for a thorough review of cognitive tools available to supplement the AAC evaluation process, as well as other key features of a thorough AAC evaluation regardless of disability.

As cited previously, often the individual with ASD may begin with AAC to benefit from intensive early intervention, and as the speech-language pathologist works with the child, emerging language begins, often resulting in the use of verbal speech. A second form of dynamic assessment for AAC that may be embedded within the preliminary intervention approach is the use of the Picture Exchange Communication System (PECS, Frost and Bondy 2002), which can be used to observe pre-linguistic behaviors and early emerging skills related to competent AAC use, such as cause and effect, visual discrimination, early syntax use following a developmental sequence for oral speech, and left-to-right correspondence for emerging literacy. As treatment goals are established, the PECS system may be used to introduce the concept of AAC to the child in order to obtain desired items and activities, and to socially interact with others. Frost and Bondy (2002) report that PECS was not designed with an outcome of verbal speech as the goal; however, it is often the case that verbal speech begins to emerge when the PECS system is followed. The PECS system relies heavily on principles of applied behavior analysis, and is considered an emerging evidence-based practice within ASD interventions (National Autism Center 2015). When used with fidelity, the PECS system often results in one of two decision-making outcomes on the part of the clinician: (1) continue language development using the verbal speech modality if verbal speech has emerged or (2) continue language development using a more advanced AAC device once initial behaviors such as initiating, requesting, commenting, visual discrimination, and combining symbols have been observed with the PECS system. PECS is a low-tech AAC tool that facilitates the transition to more advanced AAC options because the system addresses the necessary pre-linguistic skills needed for AAC use and communicative competence through an explicit, sequenced hierarchy, and structured teaching approach. In addition, the key component of PECS that lends itself well to bridging skills for AAC use is the emphasis on initiating communication attempts to others. Without that essential communication skill, an AAC tool will be of little use to the child with autism. Often clinicians or parents may indicate that PECS had been tried in the past, with no success; however, it is critical to reassess the child's use of PECS taking the strict sequencing and prompting approach outlined in the system, in order to ensure it has been implemented with fidelity before assuming the system "did not work." This process can be done in a very short period of time and lays the ground work for moving the child forward with AAC that is meaningful and predictable following a similar pattern of communication the child had been trained on. Children performing at Phase 4 of the PECS system, which requires putting symbols together independently on a PECS sentence strip and initiating an exchange with a communication partner, should be able to transition to a SGD with little difficulty if the child will physically point to each symbol on a PECS strip as the communication partner reads the message out loud. If the child is not yet pointing, this behavior can be encouraged through physical prompting and positive reinforcement using preferred items and activities paired with verbal modeling (Frost and Silverman-McGowan 2014).

It is of paramount importance that in attempts to create AAC for basic communication needs throughout the child's day that clinicians not inadvertently ignore the development of more sophisticated forms of language as the child demonstrates progress with any AAC device. It is still very important that the team of professionals working with the child consider how the child is using language relative to the sequence of language development observed in typically developing children. Given a critical window for developing language, the reader is encouraged to review Brown's (1973) stages of morphological development in order to understand the complexity of the early developing language system, whether oral- or AAC-assisted. These morpho-syntactic features of language are essential in building and expanding expression and comprehension of language. The AAC must encompass the use of these morpho-syntactic features as part of its design and should allow flexibility in developing the system in accordance with the level of language development the child demonstrates. The speech-language pathologist should be consulted as the AAC system evolves in order to align with the language level of the child as these skills emerge.

AAC Tools and Technology Recently Developed to Support Communication for ASD

As the area of technology is constantly changing, new approaches to its use for AAC will grow in scope, as it applies to autism. By the time of this publication, it is feasible that a number of new developments will have been made, thus a brief overview of existing high-tech tools will be discussed to illustrate the current technology. An emerging area within the realm of augmentative alternative communication and assistive technology includes software programs and apps that capitalize on recent autism research related to visual attention and eye tracking. Innovative technologies to increase the child's response to visual stimuli have emerged with the promise of promoting increased attention to verbal speech and increased observation of socially appropriate behaviors. Just as in the case of AAC for communication, the use of these therapy tools for teaching oral speech requires that the child possess some basic pre-linguistic skills such as engagement with tasks and activities, joint attention, and initiations before implementing them. Such technology includes apps that focus on the mouth as verbal speech is successively increased through the introduction of phonemes, then to full communication messages, combining two words, then sentences, with a video model to support the teaching process. An example of this technology is the app known as Inner Voice©, which is based on empirical research related to the use of video modeling (Cardon and Azuma 2012; Charlop-Christy et al. 2000; Vivanti et al. 2008) as the basis for the AAC technology. This SGD app not only includes dynamic displays with basic icons for functional communication, but also includes the added feature of a video image of the child producing the verbal message as the message is spoken. Research in the area of video self-modeling indicates that when the child with autism observes him- or herself performing a given behavioral act, as with other forms of video modeling, the likelihood of the child exhibiting the behavior increases (Bellini and Akullian 2006; Wert and Neisworth 2003) when compared to other methods. The Inner Voice© app is also based on emerging research indicating that individuals with autism respond to intervention utilizing avatars, resulting in an increase in social interaction and emotion recognition (Hopkins et al. 2011), providing the rationale for including the option of adding an avatar or character performing the messages if desired. It has been suggested by the makers of Inner Voice© that this app may promote an increase in verbal speech, taking the focus off of the therapist for learning the communication targets, while utilizing highly motivating visual stimuli based on basic research in the area of visual processing and eye gaze in the ASD population. This area of AAC research is relatively new, and although based on empirical evidence to support the approach to gain visual attention and focus, outcomes regarding clinical trials using this specific app have yet to be completed.

Apps based on typical AAC formats and emerging research regarding VSDs are now commonly found. It is important to note that parents are often accessing these communication systems prior to having their child formally evaluated, so it is not uncommon to work with a child with autism who has had some exposure to AAC, albeit with limited structure or explicit teaching involved in the process of introducing the technology. An example of an app available to consumers utilizing a picture cell-based format is the Proloquo2Go© application, available for download on mobile devices and tablets. Proloquo2Go© is a commonly used AAC SGD which has the potential to expand vocabulary and language beyond simple communication messages. Messages are selected from symbol cell page layouts with dynamic displays and can be simplified to as few as 4 cells on a page as the child is learning to use the AAC, to more than 20 cells on a page, as the child's abilities increase. This app is more like other traditional AAC devices in its design and lends itself well to transition from a basic AAC system or low-tech system such as PECS. An example of a current SGD app built on the use of VSDs is the AutismMate©, designed to incorporate vocabulary within the context of picture scenes, and has the option of traditional cell-based page layouts. Just as with InnerVoice©, the AutismMate© capitalizes on emerging visual processing research and eye gaze data to support the foundation for AAC use and the autism population. For the three examples presented, there are a number of variations of these formats put out by other companies. In addition to apps, there still exist the more traditional dedicated AAC devices, which include the VanguardPlus©, Dynavox©, and the lower-tech, but functionally useful, GoTalk20©. Familiarity with these devices is helpful as device options are discussed. It is also important to bear in mind physical needs of the child, the potential for any damage to the type of equipment being recommended, as well as cost.

Although all of these apps and AAC options hold promise for children with ASD, the technology alone does not replace the need for specialized skill and training in the area of AAC and the need for a comprehensive evaluation of communicative behaviors. As discussed, evaluation of visual discrimination, ability to combine symbols, pointing, and use of communication initiations paired with highly motivating items and activities are necessary before introducing any form of AAC. Given the rate at which technology is evolving, a single app or AAC device by name should not be what is sought out for the child with ASD so much as attention to the evaluation process, to ensure successful transition and use of the chosen device. Additionally, existing research in the area of early intervention and essential components to early intervention programs in terms of long-term outcomes should not be ignored. In a seminal review of research that included the establishment of essential components of effective early intervention programs for ASD, Dawson and Osterling (1997) found that the inclusion of predictability and routine, paired with strong visual support, and parental involvement all yielded more positive outcomes for preschool children with ASD receiving early intervention. These same components should be considered as AAC is introduced to the child with ASD and should include education for the parent regarding treatment goals and rationale for goals, as well as ways in which the parent can promote the use of the AAC in the home through application of behavioral intervention and reinforcement for communication attempts, both pre-linguistic and language-based.

Initial Treatment Goals

Once a thorough assessment has been conducted, initial goals for introducing the AAC technology must be established based on assessment results and goals of the family. Collectively, the team develops initial targets, with the knowledge that AAC intervention with the child with autism is an ongoing form of dynamic assessment, in which the direction of its use will constantly change as the child and communication partners adapt to the AAC system. Although the needs will vary from individual to individual depending upon presenting behaviors, a typical path regarding development of initial treatment goals follows the sequence below:

(a) Initiating a communicative exchange using a 1:1 correspondence of symbol to object;
(b) Requesting a preferred item when given a choice of two symbols on the AAC;
(c) Initiating functional communicative phrases within play routines and daily activities (e.g., "My turn," "Good morning," "All done!");
(d) Matching vocabulary on the AAC device to objects within categories to build expressive vocabulary (e.g., dress, pants, shoes; truck, car, boat);
(e) Combining symbols to request (e.g., "red car," "brown crayon") and comment ("Truck go!"); and
(f) Expanding communicative partners and contexts.

The sequence described builds on the use of initiations, visual discrimination, and emerging use of abstract language. An emphasis on building expressive vocabulary helps the individual with autism begin to develop schema that is required in order to use more sophisticated forms of AAC. From a behavioral standpoint, developing goals related to social engagement with others, especially with multiple communicative partners in varied settings, is a critical step in the use of AAC. The child with ASD will quickly learn that the use of the AAC provides a sense of control and predictability, when others respond in the same way to the use of the AAC. Emotions, and basic wants and needs related to self-help, should also be incorporated into the basic vocabulary, but must also be taught in explicit, concrete terms.

Data collection with careful consideration of prompting and fading of cues is also a critical step in the introduction of AAC. The goal is independent use of the AAC, and an increase in the use of pre-linguistic behaviors to support its use without dependence on an adult.

Why AAC Often Fails or Becomes Minimally Supportive for Communication

This chapter provides a framework for developing an evaluation of communication and language needs that is comprehensive and guides the development of initial treatment goals relative to AAC use. Although specific AAC options have been discussed, the options shared are broad-based examples of various forms of AAC currently used with the ASD population and should not be considered exhaustive of all options. The basic premise of thorough evaluation and specific targeting of pre-linguistic behaviors to yield more productive AAC use guides the clinician in understanding why AAC may not be working for the individual with ASD. Lack of success with AAC use may be the result of: (i) introducing the AAC too early or prior to the development of fundamental pre-linguistic behaviors, (ii) lack of intentional sequencing of teaching communicative behaviors and subsequent combination of communication symbols using the device chosen, or (iii) lack of identifying communicative contexts that promote the use of the device with both familiar and unfamiliar communication partners based on daily routines and meeting wants and needs.

When determining the initial stages of developing the communication page layout, one should bear in mind that following a typical sequence for oral language should apply with the AAC as well. For example, teaching the child to point, use single-word vocabulary and one-to-one correspondence with a symbol and object, then begin to combine two "words" or symbols, follows a typical pattern of oral language development in typical children, and allows expansion of language skill in the AAC user. Often this path of acquiring language is ignored by providers, and icons are randomly presented based on preferred objects and immediate needs only. In addition to purposely designing the language capability, the AAC team serving the child with ASD should work to identify and contrive specific opportunities that require the child to use the device and build on success as the child begins to show communicative competence. Beukelman and Mirenda (2013) is an excellent resource for teams seeking out templates to guide the development of these contexts in daily interactions with the AAC user. Attention to behavioral reinforcement should also be considered as AAC is introduced. In the case of autism, often undesirable forms of communication, specifically unconventional means of communication such as screaming or hitting, may be reinforced by others as opposed to differential reinforcement of other behaviors that are more appropriate. In this case, if the AAC is not being used, it is essential that the team analyze the behaviors that are occurring and determine ways to differentially reinforce the desired behavior, which is using the device to communicate, as opposed to hitting or screaming to get needs met. In a case such as this, a functional behavioral analysis (FBA) may be helpful. Last, a common reason the AAC device may not be successful with the child with ASD may be due to the chosen technology, which may not be in alignment with the neurologic behaviors and cognitive ability of the child. Based on this brief review of neuroscience research related to visual processing and analysis of cognitive skills necessary to use various forms of AAC, assessment tools have been referenced to help teams avoid this error. If an advanced AAC option has already been selected by the parent, the supportive clinician may encourage a family to scaffold to a temporary device option that more closely matches the needs of the child as initial goals are developed. In this case, education to the parent, as well as providing a rationale for AAC choice, should be given. Parents should be given training on promoting optimal use of the AAC in the form of hands-on support as the parent interacts with the child, and through the use of video demonstration of interaction with the speech-language pathologist and other communicative partners.

A New Era in ASD Intervention and Hope for the Future

To summarize, thorough evaluation of pre-linguistic behaviors is necessary before implementing AAC, transitioning from low-tech to high-tech options may be prudent in most cases, and consideration of the neural challenges associated with

ASD, such as eye gaze, visual attention, and visual discrimination, should be considered as part of a thorough assessment when introducing AAC technology.

As technology continues to advance in the area of AAC, and as our understanding of the ASD brain evolves, there is hope for meeting the communication needs of this population, and there is hope for the families in relating to their children in new ways. Given the promising preliminary results of early intervention outcome data related to ASD intervention, paired with innovative technological advances for ease of use and access to tools for communication, the next decade offers a new era in ASD research and examination of treatment efficacy related to AAC use. Collaboration among professionals is the key for promoting the most optimal outcomes as AAC is addressed, and operating from the understanding that each discipline offers specific expertise in the ongoing analysis of treatment outcomes related to the AAC use is essential to ensure success.

References

Amaral, D., Schumann, C. M., & Nordahl, C. (2008). Neuroanatomy of autism. *Trends in Neurosciences, 31*(3), 137–145.

American Psychiatric Association. (2013). *Diagnostic and statistical manual of mental disorders* (5th ed.). Washington, DC: Author.

American Speech-Language Hearing Association. (2014). *Augmentative and alternative communication*. Washington, DC: Author. Retrieved from: http://www.asha.org/public/speech/disorders/AAC/.

American Speech-Language-Hearing Association. (2004). *Roles and responsibilities of speech-language pathologists with respect to augmentative and alternative communication: technical report*. Retrieved from: www.asha.org/policy.

Apple, Inc. (2105). *I-Pad software*. Cupertino, CA. Retrieved from: https://www.apple.com/ipad/.

Bellini, S., & Akullian, J. (2006). A meta-analysis of video modeling and video self-modeling interventions for children and adolescents with autism spectrum disorders. *Exceptional Children, 73*(3), 264–287.

Beukelman, D., & Mirenda, P. (2013). *Augmentative and alternative communication. Supporting children and adults with complex communication needs* (4th ed.). Baltimore, MD: Brookes.

Brown, R. (1973). *A first language: The early stages*. London: George Allen & Unwin.

Cardon, T., & Azuma, (2012). Visual attending preferences in children with autism spectrum disorders: A comparison between live and video presentation modes. *Research in Autism Spectrum Disorders, 6*(3), 1061–1067.

Centers for Disease Control and Prevention. (2014). *Autism: Research*. Atlanta, GA: Author.

Charlop-Christy, M. H., Le, L., & Freeman, K. A. (2000). A comparison of video modeling with in vivo modeling for teaching children with autism. *Journal of Autism and Developmental Disorders, 30*(6), 537–552.

Dawson, G. (2008). Early behavioral intervention, brain plasticity, and the prevention of autism spectrum disorder. *Development and Psychopathology, 20*(3), 775–803.

Dawson, G., & Osterling, J. (1997). Early intervention in autism. In M. Guralnick (Ed.), *The effectiveness of early intervention* (pp. 307–326). Baltimore, MD: Paul H. Brookes Publishing.

Dawson, G., Rogers, S., Munson, J., Smith, M., Winter, J., Greenson, J., et al. (2010). Randomized, controlled trial of an intervention for toddlers with autism: The Early Start Denver Model. *Pediatrics, 125*, 17–24.

Dynavox. (2014). *Dynavox, Mayer-Johnson*. Pittsburgh, PA. Retrieved from: http://www. dynavoxtech.com/company/contact/.

Fisher, W., Piazza, C., Bowman, L., Hagopian, L. P., Owens, J. C., & Slevin, I. (1992). A comparison of two approaches for identifying reinforcers for persons with severe and profound disabilities. *Journal of Applied Behavior Analysis, 25*, 491–498.

Frost, L., & Bondy, A. (2002). *The picture exchange communication system training manual* (2nd ed.). Pyramid Educational Consultants, Inc.

Frost, L., & Silverman-McGowan, J. (2014). Strategies for transitioning from PECS to SGD, part 2: Maintaining communication competency. *Perspectives on Augmentative and Alternative Communication.* Retrieved from: http://sig12perspectives.pubs.asha.org.

Gillespie-Smith, K., & Fletcher-Watson, S. (2014). Designing AAC systems for children with autism: Evidence from eye tracking research. *Augmentative and Alternative Communication.* doi:10.3109/07434618.2014.905635.

Hadjikhani, N., Joseph, R. M., Snyder, J., Chabris, C., Clark, J., Steele, S., et al. (2004). Activation of the fusiform gyrus when individuals with autism spectrum disorder view faces. *Neuroimage, 22*(3), 1141–1150.

Hartley, S.L., Barker, E.T., Seltzer, M.M., Floyd, F., Greeburg, J., Orsmond, G, & Bolt, D. (2010). The relative risk and timing of divorce in families of children with an autism spectrum disorder. *Journal of Family Psychology,, 24*(4), 449–457.

Helt, M., Kelley, E., Kinsbourne, M., Pandey, J., Boorstein, H., Herbert, M., et al. (2008). Can children with autism recover? If so, how? *Neuropsychology Review, 18*(4), 339–366.

Hernandez, N., Metzger, A., Magne, R., Bonnet-Brilhault, F., Roux, S., Barthelemy, C., & Martineau, J. (2009). Exploration of core features of a human face by healthy and autistic adults analyzed by visual scanning. *Neuropsychologia, 47*, 1004–1012.

Hopkins, I. M., Gower, M. W., Perez, T. A., Smith, D. S., Amthor, F. R., Winsatt, F. C., & Biasini, F. J. (2011). Avatar assistant: Improving social skills in students with an ASD through a computer-based intervention. *Journal of Autism and Developmental Disorders, 41*(11), 1543–1555.

Kaderavek, J. N. (2011). *Language disorders in children: Fundamental concepts of assessment and intervention*. Boston, MA: Pearson Education.

Koegel, R. L., & Koegel, L. K. (2006). *Pivotal response treatments for autism: communication, social, and academic development*. Baltimore, Md.: Paul H. Brookes Publishing.

Le Couteur, A., Lord, C., & Rutter, M. (2003). *Autism diagnostic interview-revised. Manual.* Torrance, CA: Western Psychological Services.

Lord, C., Rutter, M., DiLavore, P., & Risi, S. (2001). *Autism diagnostic observation schedule. Manual.* Los Angeles, CA: Western Psychological Services.

Mailick Seltzer, M., Greenberg, J. S., Hong, J., Smith, L. E., Almeida, D. M., Coe, C., et al. (2009). Maternal cortisol levels and behavior problems in adolescents and adults with ASD. *Journal of Autism and Developmental Disorders, 40*(4), 457–469.

Mesibov, G. B., Shea, V., Schopler, E., Adams, L., Merkler, E., Burgess, S., et al. (2004). *The TEACCH approach to autism spectrum disorders*. US: Springer.

Meyer-Johnson (2014). *GoTalk20*. Pittsburgh, PA. Retrieved from: http://www.mayer-johnson. com/gotalk-20.

Mirenda, P. (2014). Autism spectrum disorder, past, present, future. *Perspectives.* Retrieved from: http://sig12perspectives.pubs.asha.org/ on 02/03/2014.

Mirenda, P., Smith, I. M., Volden, J., Szatmari, P., Bryson, S., Fombonne, E., et al. (2013). *How many children with autism spectrum disorder are functionally nonverbal?* Paper presented at the International Meeting for Autism Research, San Sebastian, Spain.

National Academy of Sciences-National Research Council. (2001). *Educating children with autism.* Washington DC: Author.

National Autism Center. (2015). *Findings and Conclusions: National standards project, Phase 2. Addressing the need for evidence-based practice guidelines for autism spectrum disorders.* Randolph, MA: National Autism Center.

Pelphrey, K. A., Sasson, N. J., Reznick, J. S., Paul, G., Goldman, B. D., & Piven, J. (2002). Visual scanning of faces in autism. *Journal of Autism and Developmental Disorders, 32*, 249–261.

Piaget, J. (1953). *The origin of intelligence in the child*. New Fetter Lane, New York: Routledge & Kegan Paul.

Prentke-Romich Company. (2015). *Vanguard Plus*. Wooster, OH. Retrieved from: https://www.prentrom.com/support/category/6.

Prizant, B., Wetherby, A., Rubin, E., Laurent, A., & Rydell, P. (2006). *The SCERTS model: A comprehensive educational approach for children with autism spectrum disorders*. Baltimore, MD: Paul H. Brookes Publishing.

Riby, D. M., & Hancock, P. J. B. (2009). Do faces capture the attention of individuals with Williams Syndrome or autism? Evidence from tracking eye movements. *Journal of Autism and Developmental Disorders, 39*, 421–431.

Rogers, S. J., & Dawson, G. (2009). *Early start denver model for young children with autism*. New York, NY: Guilford Press.

Rowland, C. (1996, 2004). *Communication matrix*. Portland, OR: Design to Learn.

Schopler, E., & Van Bourgondien, M. E. (2010). *Childhood autism rating scale* (2nd ed.). Los Angeles, CA: Western Psychological Services.

SpecialNeedsWare. (2014). *AutismMate*. Retrieved from: http://specialneedsware.com/About-SpecialNeedsWare/Advisors/.

van der Meer, L., Sutherland, D., O'Reilly, M. F., Lancioni, G. E., & Sigafoos, J. (2012). A further comparison of manual signing, picture exchange, and speech-generating devices as communication modes for children with autism spectrum disorders. *Research in Autism Spectrum Disorders, 6*(4), 1247–1257.

Vivanti, G., Nadig, A., Ozonoff, S., & Rogers, S. J. (2008). What do children with autism attend to during imitation tasks? *Journal of Experimental Child Psychology, 101*(3), 186–205.

Wert, B. Y., & Neisworth, J. T. (2003). Effects of video self-modeling on spontaneous requesting in children with autism. *Journal of Positive Behavior Interventions, 5*(1), 30–34.

Wilkinson, K. M., & Light, J. (2014). Preliminary study of eye gaze toward humans in photographs by individuals with autism, down syndrome, or other intellectual disabilities: Implications for design of visual scene displays. *Augmentative and Alternative Communication*. doi:10.3109/07434618.2014.904434.

Wilkinson, K. M., Light, J., & Drager, K. (2012). Considerations for the composition of visual scene displays: Potential contributions of information from visual and cognitive sciences. *Augmentative and Alternative Communication, 28*(3), 137–147.

Williams, J. H. G., Massaro, D. W., Peel, N. J., Bosseler, A., & Suddendorf, T. (2004). Visual–auditory integration during speech imitation in autism. *Research in Developmental Disabilities, 25*(6), 559–575.

World Health Organization. (2013). *Autism spectrum disorders & other developmental disorders. From raising awareness to building capacity*. Geneva, Switzerland: Author.

Chapter 3
The Use of Technology in the Treatment of Autism

Kristie Brown Lofland

Recent statistics released from the Center of Disease Control (CDC) indicate that in the USA, 1 out of 68 children will be diagnosed with an autism spectrum disorder (ASD). Studies indicate that 10–20% of these children will be unable to communicate their wants, needs, and thoughts verbally. According to the statistics reported by the CDC, that means over 20,000 children are born each year who will be diagnosed with ASD and remain functionally nonverbal. When individuals have severe speech and language disabilities, augmentative and alternative communication strategies (AAC) can provide them with an opportunity to express themselves and have a voice. The inability to communicate has a significant impact on the quality of life, education access, and development of social skills and relationships. The frustration of not being able to communicate can lead to behavior challenges as well.

AAC services developed from the most basic desire to help individuals who were unable to speak or express themselves to the people around them. In the earliest form, eye gaze, letter, and picture displays were included as AAC. In order to utilize these early forms, face-to-face interaction was required, and the interaction was usually slow. As microprocessor technology was developed, dedicated AAC systems were custom-built by small, dedicated AAC companies using synthesized speech. These systems were often heavy, cumbersome, and expensive. Personal computers (PC) and standard operating systems became another option for AAC and opened up a new world for developers. Not only could consumers use the technology for face-to-face interactions, but they could also use the technology to write, create, and give presentations and more readily participate in their home, school, work, and community environments. The PC devices were more portable and a little less expensive than the previous dedicated AAC devices. Then along came mobile, multiple use technologies that offered opportunities to the AAC consumer and/or learner that extended far beyond the capacity of current AAC devices and at significantly lower costs. Digital computer technology has become a

K.B. Lofland (✉)
Indiana Resource Center for Autism, Indiana University, Bloomington, IN, USA
e-mail: klofland@indiana.edu

© Springer International Publishing Switzerland 2016

T.A. Cardon (ed.), *Technology and the Treatment of Children with Autism Spectrum Disorder*, Autism and Child Psychopathology Series, DOI 10.1007/978-3-319-20872-5_3

prevalent feature of everyday life and is an increasingly popular means of communication in today's society.

The proliferation of inexpensive mobile technology has dramatically changed how service providers deliver educational and behavioral services to individuals with ASD. From touch screen phones to tablet devices, mobile computing devices have never been more user-friendly, less expensive, or universally available.

Research findings indicate that as the development of new communication technology progresses at an increasing rate each year, children's competency and awareness of such technology also inevitably increases—oftentimes overtaking that of their parents' competence. Children's increasing use of technology has implication for both educational and communicational practices, because it is now a prevalent environment factor in their lives (Watt 2010). Children today are often referred to as "native speakers" of technology. This is often true for our students with ASD. Many ASD individuals are more comfortable interacting with inanimate objects such as a computer or iPad. In addition, many individuals are visual learners and have strong technological skills.

In the past two years, there have been many "made-for-TV" commentaries highlighting the use of technology with individuals with autism. Usually, these commentaries have focused upon a child who could not communicate and often had behavioral issues due to the frustration of not being able to communicate. Once introduced to a communication app on the iPad, the child was able to communicate eloquent thoughts and inappropriate behaviors disappeared. Therefore, due to the media hype, many consumers began to purchase an iDevice and a certain communication app at an alarming rate, because they were sure that an iPad was a panacea for every individual with ASD. Like all technologies and techniques, certain things work for certain people. Not all individuals with ASD need the iPad for a communication system, but they could have used the technology to increase another skill. However, the consumer who purchased the iPad did not know how to evaluate what app to purchase, what app was appropriate, etc. Therefore, the majority of the iPads were used for entertainment and game playing. We now know that mobile technology can be used effectively for not only entertainment and as an AAC device, but to also assist in teaching academic areas, social skills, video modeling, reinforcement, ABA, speech/language therapy, fine motor skills, visual supports, functional life skills, organizational skills, and increasing independence.

People with ASD have a need for, and a right to, the same range of communication options available to everyone else. Today, most people use multiple devices to address their communication needs. The idea that only ONE communication device can meet every need no longer makes sense. Some needs may be met by the mainstream device, while others may require accessories and techniques specifically designed for them (e.g., eye gaze, scanning, adapted keyboards). Multiple use technology extends past our current AAC technology and at a significant lower cost.

A growing concern for all individuals with ASD is employment and having skills to live independently. National data indicate that the majority of adults with autism are unemployed or underemployed. Employment is a critical component for having a productive adult life. Individuals living with autism deserve the opportunity to contribute as productive workers in appropriate employment settings, paying taxes and improving their quality of life. Barriers to successful employment for individuals with autism can be poor communication skills; social "soft skills" such as small talk, office politics, and unspoken requirements; the ability to complete the job independently without a job coach; or sensory issues within the work environment. The use of mobile technology can address some of these barriers.

So Why Is Technology Helpful in Treating Individuals with ASD?

Using devices like tablets and other handheld devices are useful tools, because they are flexible and portable unlike other dedicated AAC devices that often can be heavy and cumbersome to transport. A handheld device is easily carried for on the go, and there is peer acceptance. The touch screen and layout are more accessible for individuals with coordination or learning difficulties—sliding and tapping are easier than typing. Technology can improve communication with others by the timely use of email or texting, which has a cost and time savings. Technology allows for adaptability and motivation.

Many people with ASD are visual thinkers. According to Temple Grandin, author, speaker, and an individual with ASD, pictures are their first language, and words are their second language. As concrete, literal, visual thinkers, individuals with autism can process information better when they are looking at pictures or words to help them visualize information. Technology just makes visual images more accessible to the ASD individual. Computer graphics capture and maintain their attention.

Some individuals may have auditory sensitivity and are better able to respond to lower sounds. Using computers, we can easily download appropriate voice levels and adjust sound according to the individual's needs. An individual with ASD or his/her family may use an app like *Noise Down,* which will automatically sound an alarm when the decibel level gets too high, or *Too Noisy Pro* to indicate to the individual that they are being too loud.

Some individuals with autism are unable to sequence. Technology can reduce the number of steps required for the completion of a task or give a visual representation of the task steps in sequence. An example of an app for sequencing tasks is *Sequencing Tasks: Life Skills.* Sequencing options are lists of printed words, words and pictures, just pictures, voice/no voice, etc.

Often individuals with ASD have difficulty with fine motor skills making handwriting difficult. Technology helps reduce the frustration with handwriting or drawing. Using a keyboard, touch screen, or speech-to-text app can reduce the difficulty and frustration, thus increasing the individual's enjoyment for learning. Considering the national data on employment for individuals with autism, teaching technology for skills such as writing needs to be employed as early as possible. Yes, knowing how to write your signature and other information is important, especially when technology is not available; however, when looking at what handwriting skills are currently being utilized today versus keyboarding, dictation, or writing on a screen with a stylus or your finger, we clearly see the current skills needed. In addition, there are many apps that allow individuals to practice fine motor skills in other areas besides handwriting or keyboarding.

Some individuals do not use speech for communication or, in times of high stress, need additional augmentation in producing verbal thoughts and words. They can use technology as a voice output device to speak for them and help them express themselves more fluently. Nonverbal children with autism find it easier to associate words with pictures if they see the printed words and a picture together. The Web can give unlimited access to pictures and words! There are numerous AAC apps, from low to high tech, that can be used by individuals living with autism.

It is thought that some individuals with autism cannot look and listen at the same time. Their immature sensory systems cannot process simultaneous visual and auditory input. Using technology, they can gradually increase their ability to use both or alternate between visual and auditory input.

Some children with autism will learn to read phonetically, and others will learn visually with whole words. Voice output helps with the auditory reinforcement, and computer graphics can help the students visualize the words and, therefore, increase their reading skills.

Many individuals with autism have difficulty with executive functioning and struggle with organizational and self-management skills. Again, there are several apps that will assist with organization and self-management with calendars, schedules, work systems, etc. Apps such as *Visual Schedule Planner*, *Pocket Schedule*, or *Functional Planning System* are just a few that assist with organization and self-management.

Today, there are over one million apps available, and the number continues to grow daily. The apps range in price from free to several hundred dollars. There is an app for anything and everything. However, caution must be used. Like all strategies used for the treatment of ASD, the selection of the technology and/or the apps must be personalized to meet the individual needs of the learner. Assessment and data are necessary before making a decision about any technology used. What is the population/individual you will be working with? What skills do you want to target? In what context will the technology/app be used? How do these skills compare with their peers? What will be the expected outcomes?

Two good search engines for finding appropriate apps are *Autism Apps* and *i.AM Search*. *Autism Apps* will allow you to search by category, price, and device rating for the skill/s you want to target. *Autism Apps* links to reviews by parents, specialists, and other users, usually from first-hand experience; it also has links to video demonstrations or video reviews of the app when available. *i.AM Search* allows you to create a profile for an individual by supplying the age, gender, and level of dependence of the individual on others, to the level of the individual's independent use of technology. Once the information is entered, it will do a quick search for appropriate apps fitting that profile for you to review.

Some Web sites for looking for apps are the following:

Smart apps for Special Needs
www.smartappsforspecialneeds.com/
Apps and Autism
http://www.ipodsibilities.com/iPodsibilities/AppsandAutism.html
Apps for Children with Special Needs
http://a4cwsn.com
Autism Apps
https://autismapps.wikispaces.com
Mobile Learning 4 Special Needs
https://mobilelearning4specialneeds.wikispaces.com

When looking at the evidence-based practices for ASD which can be supported by technology, the following practices are evident: visual supports, video modeling, reinforcement, social skills, discrete trial training, self-management, social narratives, technology-assisted intervention and implementation, and task analysis.

Technology-Assisted Intervention and Implementation (TAII)

TAII is a combination of two previously identified evidence-based practices—computer-aided instruction and voice output communication aid (VOCA) or speech-generating devices (SGDs). Computer-aided instruction includes the use of computers to teach academic skills and to promote communication and language development and skills. It includes computer modeling and computer tutors. SGDs are electronic devices that are portable in nature and can produce either synthetic or digital speech for the user. SGDs may be used with graphic symbols as well as with alphabet keys.

SGDs/VOCAs can be low tech, such as a two-choice toggle switch, or can be a full-featured communication solution with over 10,000 available symbols for individuals who have difficulty using their natural voice. Two of the most popular SGDs/VOCAs are *Proloquo@Go* and *TouchChat*. Both are grid-based communication systems, meaning that they have multiple pages in a grid layout with buttons, messages, and symbols that are fully customizable.

Visual Supports

If you are a visual learner, seeing it makes all the difference, especially when it comes to students with ASD. Individuals with ASD are able to process information easier when it is visual and spatial. Spoken language tends to be abstract, transient, and temporal. While written language can also be abstract, it is less transient than verbal language. Visual supports, an evidenced-based practice for individuals with ASD, are typically used daily to enhance the individual's understanding. With visual supports, individuals with ASD can learn more quickly, reduce interfering behavior, decrease frustration and anxiety, learn to adjust to change, complete tasks by themselves, and gain independence. However, it can be very time-consuming to create drawings, images, schedules, or other visuals; to customize the materials to highlight key features; and to print and laminate them. The task of making the world more visual for individuals with ASD has evolved through the use of various apps and programs. For example, *Choiceworks* is an app that is designed for both iPhone and iPad that will help children complete daily routines, understand and control their feelings, and improve their waiting skills through the use of visual schedules, routines, and choices.

Video Modeling

Video modeling is a mode of teaching that uses video recording and display equipment to provide a visual model of the targeted behavior or skill. Types of video modeling include basic video modeling, video self-modeling, point-of-view video modeling, and video prompting. Basic video modeling involves recording someone besides the learner engaging in the target behavior or skill. The video is then viewed by the learner at a later time. Video self-modeling is used to record the learner displaying the target skill or behavior and is reviewed later. Point-of-view video modeling is when the target behavior or skill is recorded from the perspective of the learner. Video prompting involves breaking the behavior or skill into steps and recording each step with incorporated pauses during which the learner may attempt the step before viewing subsequent steps. Video prompting may be done with either the learner or someone else acting as a model. The video and camera quality and ease of use of handheld devices enable practitioners to incorporate this evidence-based practice into treatment of individuals with ASD. Research indicates that video modeling can be an effective strategy in helping individuals with autism develop social skills and daily living skills. There are currently several apps, such as *Model Me Kids,* on the market for teaching perspective taking.

Social Narratives

Social narratives are interventions that describe social situations in some detail by highlighting relevant cues and offering examples of appropriate responding. They are designed to help learners adjust to changes in routine and adapt their behaviors based on the social and physical cues of a situation, or to teach specific social skills or behaviors. Social narratives are individualized according to learner needs and typically are quite short, perhaps including pictures or other visual aids. Sentence types that are often used when constructing social narratives include descriptive, directive, perspective, affirmative, control, and cooperative. Apps that can be used to create social narratives are *Pictello*, *Story Kit*, *Story Creator*, and *My Pictures Talk*.

Reinforcement

Reinforcement describes a relationship between learner behavior and a consequence that follows the behavior. This relationship is only considered reinforcement if the consequence increases the probability that a behavior will occur in the future, or at least be maintained. For example, children learn to ask for something politely if they want to receive it in return. The ultimate goal of reinforcement is to help learners with ASD learn new skills and maintain their use over time in a variety of settings with many different individuals. As such, teachers and other practitioners must identify the appropriate reinforcers that motivate individual learners with ASD. Oftentimes, the device itself, or a particular app on the device, is a reinforcer. It is important that the individual with autism be taught that the technology has multiple uses and should not be used just for reinforcement.

A token economy program is another type of positive reinforcement strategy that can be used effectively with learners with ASD. Token economy programs are based upon a monetary system in which tokens are used to acquire a desired reinforcer. For example, learners with ASD receive tokens when they use a target skill/behavior appropriately. When learners acquire a certain number of tokens, they can be exchanged for objects or activities that are reinforcing to individual learners with ASD. An example of an app that is a token economy is *Token Board* or *123TokenMe*.

Discrete Trial Training

Discrete trial training (DTT) is a one-to-one instructional approach used to teach skills in a planned, controlled, and systematic manner. DTT is used when a learner needs to learn a skill best taught in small, repeated steps. Each trial or teaching opportunity has a definite beginning and end. Within DTT, the use of antecedents and consequences is planned and implemented. Positive praise and/or tangible rewards are used to reinforce desired skills or behaviors. Data collection is an important part of DTT and supports decision-making by providing teachers/practitioners with information about beginning skill level, progress and challenges, skill acquisition and maintenance, and generalization of learned skills or behaviors.

There are many material apps that are available for use in DTT. These materials allow for skills to be practiced across environments with both practitioners and family members. In addition, there are apps, such as *Autism DTT Pro,* which contain not only materials but also progress monitoring and charting capabilities.

In a recent study by McKinney and Vazquez (2014), participants who were delivering DTT to students with autism received audio feedback comments from their trainer on the instruction being delivered simultaneously using Bug in the Ear (BIE) devices. They were also provided with a self-study manual. The participants indicated that the use of the BIE technology helped them learn an important skill (DTT) that could be used when working with students with autism. They also indicated that the combination of the self-study manual with BIE was more effective than the self-study manual alone. Given the outcomes of the study and the mobility of technology such as BIE, technology can be used to improve a practitioner's skills in teaching DTT (or any other strategy) and to ensure that implementation fidelity is maintained. Technology in the treatment of autism can be utilized by both the individual with autism and the practitioner.

Self-management

Self-management interventions help learners with ASD learn to independently regulate their own behaviors and act appropriately in a variety of home-, school-, and community-based situations. With these interventions, learners with ASD are taught to discriminate between appropriate and inappropriate behaviors, accurately monitor and record their own behaviors, and reward themselves for behaving appropriately. As learners with ASD become more fluent with the self-management system, some of the implementation responsibilities shift from teachers, families, and other practitioners to the learners themselves. As mentioned before, software and apps are available that assist individuals with ASD to be more organized, manage their schedule in a timely manner, etc. In addition, there are apps that will also assist with self-regulation of emotions, anxiety, and social skills.

TeachMate365 or *AutisMate365* are two apps that were designed by Special Needs Ware. They are comprehensive life and learning platforms that utilize personalized visual supports to build independence, self-management, and communication skills simultaneously. Most AAC devices and apps are grid-based systems that allow children with autism to build sentences using grids of symbols to explain their needs and wants. More recently, visual scene display augmentative and alternative communication apps have emerged that allow parents and caretakers to build scenes of familiar environments and make them interactive by creating hot spots for requesting wants and needs. Visual scene display augmentative and alternative communication apps are gaining popularity in classrooms for two primary reasons. One reason is that the latest augmentative and alternative communication research shows that young children and individuals with autism have required minimal, if any, instruction before using devices configured with visual scene displays to communicate. The second reason is that visual scenes can be personalized to each user's life experiences, allowing them to engage with others on a personal level. Both apps are grid based and scene based. A picture is taken of a scene from the individual's home, school, or community and downloaded onto the screen. Hot spots are created on that scene that allow the individual to make choices via a grid-based communication system and also trigger embedded video modeling recordings, social narratives, schedules, step-by-step directions of tasks, superimposed timers, first-then boards, and a host of other visual and auditory supports. Several of the evidence-based practices are implemented within the one app. Downloading classroom-ready visual supports from the interactive content library saves time and allows for collaboration with a global community of professionals.

Summary

The decision-making process of how and when to use technology with an individual with ASD should be a thoughtful process. A decision made by a team of professionals, family members, and the individual wherein the strengths, communication needs, personal characteristics, and goals of the individual match the features of the technology. When assessing an individual for a mobile device or communication app, issues such as usability, integration, discontinuance, technology compatibility, context, and sensory and cognitive demands need to be considered. In particular, the goal of AAC has always been about communication and not about the device. The pace of technology is changing more rapidly than ever before and will continue next year, and the next, and the next. This kind of readily accessible technology is exciting and holds promises for individuals with ASD and other disabilities. There is research to be done, consumer input to be gathered, and commitments to be made. Our work in the world of autism is always evolving!

References

McKinney, T., & Vasquez, E. (2014). There's a bug in your ear!: Using technology to increase the accuracy of DTT implementation. *Education and Training in Autism and Developmental Disabilities, 49*, 594–600.

Watt, Helen J. (2010). How does the Use of Moder Communication Technology Influence Language and Literacy Developement? A Review. *Contemporary Issues in Communication Science and Disorders*, 37, 141–148

www.autismspeaks.com.

www.autismpdc.fpg.unc.edu.

www.aac-rerc.psu.edu.

www.asha.org.

Chapter 4
Technology, Autism, and Occupational Therapy

Kristi A. Jordan

Occupational therapists, working with individuals with autism spectrum disorder throughout all stages of life, use technology as a means to accomplish a wide variety of meaningful and functional activities. This includes the use of technology as a communication device, as an assistive device, as an adaptation and modification for motor skills difficulties, for academic and work skill acquisition, to teach and assist in organizational skills, and in pursuit of leisure activities. Technology is additionally used in context of behavioral interventions, as a reinforcement activity, as a visual model, as a prompt, and as a tool for promoting desired behaviors. Technology offers the ability to use a combination of universally designed and independently focused tools to remove barriers to independence and to improve participation in activities related to the domains of daily living. Occupational therapy is a diverse profession, likely due to the fact that it was historically founded by a group of individuals who worked in diverse professional backgrounds. Occupational therapy is a practice that focuses on an individual's ability to participate in or perform skills and tasks related to daily living, work, and play/leisure. Typically, an occupational therapist works with individuals who have physical, mental, or developmental issues that are impacting their ability to perform skills and to achieve independence. Occupational therapy interventions are centered on individuals and the activities that they perform as a part of their daily life. The occupational therapist analyzes tasks and task demands and then adapts the task, tools, or environment in order to allow individuals to achieve successful participation in and performance of those tasks. Those tasks that are meaningful to the individual are considered their daily "occupations."

When working with individuals with autism spectrum disorder throughout their life span, occupational therapists address core deficit areas and differences. Using physical and psychosocial theoretical approaches, occupational therapists are involved in analyzing activities requiring an individual to integrate or use motor skills, sensory motor skills, cognition, communication, social skills, behavior, and daily living or functional skills.

K.A. Jordan (✉)
OTR, Indiana Resource Center for Autism, Indiana University, Bloomington, IN, USA
e-mail: krijorda@indiana.edu

© Springer International Publishing Switzerland 2016
T.A. Cardon (ed.), *Technology and the Treatment of Children with*
Autism Spectrum Disorder, Autism and Child Psychopathology Series,
DOI 10.1007/978-3-319-20872-5_4

37

What is meaningful and functional for one individual may not be for another. Meaning and function varies with personality differences and circumstances and is also affected by life span, social and cultural differences, gender differences, and other factors. Determining that an activity has meaning and is functional to the individual is the core of the occupational therapy treatment approach.

Today's educational and therapeutic models in occupational therapy embrace diversity. Individuals have different physical needs, characteristics, backgrounds, cultures, personalities, emotional needs, cognitive abilities, experiences, learning styles, interests, social skills, physical abilities, family and social supports, and medical histories. Thus, a "one-size approach" does not fit all individuals, including those on the autism spectrum (Gregory and Chapman 2013). This model is known, in education, as differentiated instruction. Differentiated instruction is a teaching theory that is based on the idea that teaching has to vary and adapt to diverse learners, which requires flexibility in teaching, and encourages educators to modify programs or curriculum to meet individual needs, rather than modifying individuals to meet the program or curriculum. The purpose of this approach is to maximize individual success.

The three elements of differentiated instruction are applicable, not only in the educational setting, but also in therapy and home settings as they apply to activities of daily living. Information and materials presented to the individual should be accessible to them and aligned to their goals for therapy, education, and life. The process of implementing any new learning in all environments must be flexible and managed well by the therapist or by the person helping with the learning process. The challenge of whatever is being learned must be set at the right level in order to promote learning. If the task or information is already mastered or too difficult, then the challenge is not correctly matched. Continually reassessing what the individual has learned is important as this guides the process and growth that occurs. When determining what is considered a successful intervention, it is important for occupational therapists to engage and motivate individuals and involve choice-making (Gregory and Chapman 2013).

Universal Design

The importance of accessibility for all is equally paramount in the field of occupational therapy. Designing the environment, and materials within it, to be accessible, regardless of physical, emotional, or cognitive barriers, allows individuals to overcome and find success in their daily activities. Universal Design for learning was inspired by the American with Disabilities Act (ADA). This is best seen through the inclusion of curb cuts on sidewalks, which allows all individuals to equally access sidewalks and curbs within communities. Curb cuts were intended to provide accessibility to individuals in wheelchairs, but improved accessibility for all.

Universal Design supports the principles of providing multiple and flexible methods of presentation for learning, providing multiple and flexible methods of expression and apprenticeships in learning, and providing multiple and flexible options for engagement in learning.

Providing technological options allows occupational therapists to differentiate the therapeutic learning process and to universally design the adaptations for individuals. The therapist uses technology to more easily offer choices within the context of therapy and to adjust treatment in accordance with priorities and progress. Technology promotes accessibility when thoughtfully designed and planned.

When using Universal Design in choosing adaptions, it is important for the occupational therapist to consider the input of the strategies and materials used; the output, or ways to demonstrate knowledge and skill; the desired length of demonstration/performance; the difficulty of performance of skills; the expectations; and the amount of support that will be required for success (Cole et al. 2000).

It is essential, when choosing the types of adaptations or technology to use with an individual, to determine his/her learning style. Occupational therapists can create a learning profile based on formal, informal, and opportunity-based assessments. Review of records and history allows a therapist to gain information from an individual's life, including previously provided services. Individuals may have a variety of sensory learning styles such as auditory, visual, tactile or kinesthetic, or a combination of these. They may demonstrate different types of intelligence or skill that lends them to successful use of low or high technological devices and adaptations (Gregory and Chapman 2013).

Individuals on the spectrum are often visual learners and thus benefit from visual, tactile, and kinesthetic learning opportunities. Presenting information visually in a consistent and predictable manner allows the individual to process information concretely and to develop routines for both learning and response.

Cognition/Executive Functioning

One occupational performance area that benefits from the use of technology is the skill of organization for work, home, and play. The use of technology aids individuals in remembering steps and prioritizing tasks and information for daily living. This may include managing daily calendars, task lists, and retrieving information not managed by memory. Individuals may use personal information manager programs, such as Microsoft Outlook, iCal, or Google Calendar, to manage calendars, appointments, reminders, emails, and task lists. They may also use apps, word processing software or auditory prompting or recording features to remember important information (Kluth and Danaher 2010). For accessibility, VoiceOver technology allows individuals who have dyslexia or low vision to hear or "read a screen" through the text to speech adaptation. Another adaptation that allows speech to be interpreted is commonly available through the use of iOS smartphones—a program called Siri. Siri can be used to set appointments and reminders through a simple voice command. Siri allows individuals to simply use their voice to send messages, schedule meetings, place phone calls, and schedule reminders. Siri responds both verbally and visually and is customizable. Siri is able to interpret many common phrases and speech and responds to a variety of requests, such as locating places on a map or nearby events.

Email reminders and calendar reminders help with the executive functioning difficulties that may persist due to a cognitive or developmental disability. These can be set up per event or on a repeating schedule for events that occur regularly. The visual component of a pop-up reminder on the screen requires the individual to physically respond to the upcoming event which increases awareness of the priority and importance of the event. These reminders can be set to sync between any device using the same software or system. They can also be shared with others through an electronic invitation.

Disorganization may challenge those with executive functioning difficulties, but use of technology to create electronic filing systems allows individuals to keep track of and easily manage large amounts of information. By teaching an individual to create subject-specific folders, it is easier to file and manage documents and information, similar to a binder and folder system.

Team or family accountability and communication can also be a positive outcome of using an electronic system. Automatic email reminders can be set for family or support staff members to help organize and support an individual. The use of email, Web pages, and online grading systems allows schools and families closer communication throughout the school day. This provides needed information to help an individual stay organized with assignments. This communication can also be a way to facilitate communication between a parent and child when trying to discover what happened on a given school day.

Electronic task lists, using a combination of words and visuals, can help individuals to break down and complete tasks of daily living or tasks related to work and leisure more effectively. This process of task analysis is another evidence-based practice. Task analysis is the process of breaking a skill into smaller steps to make performance possible (Franzone 2009). Other practices, such as reinforcement, video modeling, or time delay, should be combined with task analysis to help the individual learn the smaller steps. As the smaller steps are mastered, the learner becomes more and more independent in his/her ability to perform the larger skill. Continued availability of the visual list after the task is mastered can also be helpful to support task completion.

Simple task lists are available in most personal information managers, such as Microsoft Office. These applications allow individuals to create schedule-based tasks within a calendar or to create a simple to-do list. Tasks can be individually assigned or can be shared by others with email or document sharing.

Sensory Issues and Technology

Occupational therapists are often involved in planning sensory activities and strategies to assist individuals on the spectrum in self-regulation, focus, and the process of learning. This may be in the form of either low-tech or high-tech adaptations. One example is the use of visual adaptions in lighting, color, or contrast when using devices to improve visual attention or perception. Use of projectors, document cameras, and 1:1 device programs in schools allows individuals visual access to information being presented.

Technology also allows for tactile accommodation by reducing frustration with tasks, such as handwriting. Some individuals with autism and related developmental differences find the sound and feel of writing on paper to be aversive and prefer using a touch screen or a keyboard for written expression (Kluth and Danaher 2010). Use of a touch screen stylus reduces friction and allows individuals to write without unpleasant sensory input. Individuals also have a variety of other options, such as using traditional, on-screen, or adapted keyboards to type information. They have the option of using dictation or speech-to-text features, to reduce tactile input when working on writing activities. Programs, such as MacSpeech Dictate or Dragon Naturally Speaking, can be installed to allow individuals to use their voice to generate text. Some of these programs also allow the individual to navigate within their operating system or device using speech. For those with tactile issues and communication difficulty, the use of voice output software on a touchpad allows accommodation for both, simultaneously.

Technology provides the ability to reduce or increase auditory stimuli. It has been found, through research, that external sounds affect learning. In fact, some studies have pointed to specific impairments in overall health and even cognitive development related to external sounds, such as airplane noise and traffic noises outside of schools (Stansfeld et al. 2005). Technology to reduce distracting noise through music or white noise via headphones, iPod, iPhone, or computer can help some individuals focus. For some students, the inability to modulate and filter out unnecessary background noises can have an impact on their attention, memory, and cognition overall. For others, additional auditory sensory input improves their ability to learn and attend to tasks. There are many tools and strategies available to achieve this. Use of digital and audio books allows individuals the extra sensory input of listening to books while reading. To increase auditory stimulation, microphones and sound amplification systems are another technological advancement that are more readily available in today's classroom. USB and wireless microphones and FM systems are now available via computers and tablets for ease of access in classrooms.

For provision of sensory activities and diets, there are specific programs and activities that have been developed using special software. These programs provide visuals and directions for sensory diets and activities. Individuals can use these specialized programs, such as the program Brain Works or SticKids, to develop a schedule of activities. Gwen Wild, the occupational therapist who developed

Brainworks, used a combination of visual supports, software, and sensory integration theory to create her product. Brainworks is available as an app or as a physical/printed program with folders, Velcro, and removable icons. SticKids is another example of sensory programming using software. This software allows a therapist to create printable, customizable schedules, and planners to be used in schools and at home. Additionally, this program is designed to facilitate data tracking. Another app, SensoryTreat, allows therapists to create sensory diet schedules using an app and is available online at http://www.sensorytreat.com/.

Videos, apps, and computer software provide opportunities to pair movement with learning and can engage the learner through virtual activities. Many schools and rehabilitation facilities have recently incorporated video game systems and activities, such as the X-box Kinect and Nintendo Wii. Games such as Wii Sports engage individuals in activities through movement. Most can also be completed with less accurate motor movements than the actual activity, which allows an individual to experience success with more challenging games or sports.

A visual option is the MeMoves video systems, which are available on DVD and online. MeMoves uses music, movement, and images for physical movement activities. This is often used for leisure, to encouragement movement, or as reinforcement for completing undesirable activities. Individuals can bowl, golf, and play a variety of sports without leaving the room. Many individuals on the spectrum find technology to be a preferred leisure activity. Playing video games, watching movies, playing on the computer, and using the Internet are often chosen activities that can take up a considerable amount of time. Using these preferred activities is a motivating way to engage the learner in what is being taught. Technology naturally becomes a reinforcing activity for desired behavior.

Communication

The importance of developing a reliable form of communication is a fundamental need of many individuals on the spectrum. Occupational therapists often serve as a team member in school or healthcare settings alongside speech therapists, to assist in determining the most effective technological device to be used for communication. Other team members that may be involved in this process are speech therapy assistants, occupational therapy assistants, special education teachers, classroom teachers, physical therapists, physical therapy assistants, paraprofessionals, general education teachers, parents, and the individual, whenever possible.

Historically, specifically devoted devices were purchased and used for communication. These devices could be relatively expensive, and choosing the correct device was often difficult. The device had to be selected based on the skill deficits and abilities, cognition, portability, cost, and function or purpose. Devices ranged from eye gaze monitors for motor impairment to switch/button style devices, and even more involved software systems that included a variety of choices. Consideration of motor skills difficulties would determine the type of switch or interface that was needed. Today, the addition of communication apps on tablets or touch screen devices provides a variety of options. To learn more about technology and communication, see Chapter.

Academics

Technology has changed today's classroom. Schools are beginning to use the aforementioned Universal Design framework to promote accessibility for all individuals. Universal Design promotes providing accessible learning materials in an accessible environment. Accessible learning materials are educational materials that can be used by all students. Being accessible means that both the content of the material and the technology used to deliver the material are accessible. Devices used, such as e-books, laptops, touch screen devices, and phones, must have the capability of providing the same materials to all learners. Occupational therapists in the school are engaged in the process of evaluating the barriers that exist for individuals in the school and in selecting devices and materials that remove those barriers. They, then, train students and staff in the technology chosen. Occupational therapists further assess and provide therapy to develop the motor skills needed for using a keyboard, mouse, or other accessible form of written communication.

Classrooms are also becoming increasingly connected to social media. Through Facebook, Instagram, Twitter, and similar sites, schools are able to dynamically promote their curriculum, activities, and communication. Parents, students, and community members can learn about school events in real time and dialogue about the subject matter in a way that is relevant. Occupational therapists become a part of this process by ensuring that students are able to access devices, and view and respond to materials and information through accommodation and adaptation.

For individuals on the spectrum, social media can be another arena for social difficulties. Occupational therapists work with teachers, parents, and school staff to address social skills differences that may surface through the use of social media, such as bullying, overexposure, and Internet safety. These issues can be addressed through social skills groups, direct services, training, and consultation.

Work Skill Acquisition

To develop skills for today's workplace, individuals have to be familiar with basic forms of technology. Most entry-level jobs require a basic understanding of technology. As the job skills and demands increase, faster-paced electronic communication and work are expected. Individuals must generally be proficient in word processing, basic data and spreadsheet programs, online file sharing, and Internet-based programs. In some cases, proficiency with additional programs, specific to the job or field, is also expected. Most companies use personal information systems or a combination of Web-based and email communication. Even the process of applying for a job has become an Internet-based process, requiring individuals to access and interface with technology. Individuals must be able to access the Internet, complete online resumes, submit professional documentation, convert files and documents, and upload files and documents required for application. Occupational therapists and educational staff often work with individuals as a part of their transition from high school to college on developing these technological skills.

Behavior

Because activities involving technology are often preferred by individuals for leisure, this interest makes use of technology naturally reinforcing and motivating. The use of technology in evidence-based practices, such as the behavioral interventions of reinforcement, results in a higher rate of performance in non-preferred activities. The Premack Principle, defined by Premack (1965), is built on this premise that pairing a non-preferred activity with a preferred activity results in a higher rate of desired behavior. Individuals may follow this principle using a "first, then" visual, earning a choice of activities after completing work. Often, the choice is related to the use of a computer or technological device or an activity related to the use of technology. Individuals may also use a token economy system on a device, which awards a symbolic reinforcement that will later be exchanged for a physical or tangible reward of choice.

Additional behavioral strategies using visual reminders and similar positive behavior supports are often used within home and classroom environments. Use of technology in creating, implementing, and communicating these reminders is dependent on the device being used, programs available, and on the ability of the individual to understand, comprehend, and follow the process being taught.

Another strategy for behavior management is to teach the practice of self-management. With self-management, individuals learn how to self-monitor their own behavior in order to increase desired behaviors and/or decrease interfering behaviors. In order to self-monitor their own behavior, they must utilize a given method to record their own performance and then receive a form of reinforcement for achieving the goal of performance. It is important for the individual to know what is expected, to be trained in the methods, and then to be coached to a level of independence within the system. Often individuals use devices considered low tech, such as clickers, token boards, or objects, and marks to track frequency of behavior. They may also use timers to measure intervals or time elapse with behaviors. Many timers and token boards are available to help manage behavior and to encourage time management and transition. In addition to low-tech options, such as the use of a standard clock or a kitchen timer, there are also computer and app-based electronic timers that can be used to indicate passage of a given time interval. Use of high-tech timers allows individuals to self-monitor while using the same device for other functions. The actual device being used will display a running time and/or set a warning and reminder about the time allotted (Busick and Neitzel 2009). One example of a visual timer that is available as a physical timer or as an app is the Time Timer. http://itunes.apple.com/us/app/time-timer/id332520417?mt=8.

Technology is more widely used in the home and classroom for behavior management and data collection. Behavior management and data collection systems allow classroom parents, teachers, and individuals to easily track behavioral data throughout the day. Data can be displayed on personal devices, the classroom interactive whiteboard, and on printouts that can be in the form of electronic or paper charts. Systems often have chart and table data that can easily be created from the saved data, allowing staff, individuals, and family members to monitor behavior and outcomes in a clear visual format. Being able to visualize performance allows individuals to self-monitor and make adjustments based on the concrete information that visual feedback provides. The visualization of data also helps parents and teachers to know what is occurring behaviorally, how often, and how much. An example of a widely used program for behavior tracking is Class Dojo, which is available at https://www.classdojo.com/.

Visual Supports involve using videos, pictures, and visual models to demonstrate what is expected. Visual supports can be used to improve task completion, particularly with independent performance. They can be used for play, work, and social activities (Hume 2008). Aforementioned task analysis strategies can be visual supports, along with behavior tracking systems and schedules.

An example of how to use this evidence-based method is through the use of video modeling. To implement video modeling, a video of the desired behavior is made and reviewed with the individual who is on the autism spectrum. The video may include the individual or may show another person performing the skill. The skill may be performed in its entirety or may be broken down into the steps, as in the practice of task analysis (Franzone and Collet-Klingenberg 2008). Video modeling is effective in combination with social skills training and can be combined with the practice of using social narratives and visual supports. Social narratives are traditionally written using a computer and printed as a handout. They can be created using the concept of video modeling, using video and audio software, and can be dubbed via audio recording over the video being viewed. Text for social narratives may also be added using captioning or text overlay in the video-editing program. By using technology to create these video models, individuals are able to visualize, plan for, and respond to the expectations more effectively. Several options of video-based social skills instructions exist, including TeachTown, Social Thinking Curriculum, and Model Me Kids. For more information on video modeling, please see Chap. 8.

Technology has become the culture into which today's individuals are born, whether they are viewed as "neurotypical" or diagnosed with an autism spectrum disorder or other neurological differences. As this generation is raised in the digital age, those who are comfortable and fluent in the use of information and technology are able to access information and the world around them. Technology offers individuals the opportunity to use a combination of universally designed or independently focused tools to remove barriers to independence and to improve participation in activities related to the domains of daily living. Occupational therapists promote technology to allow individuals to achieve successful participation in and performance of those tasks that are meaningful to the individual and thus are the occupation of their daily life.

Resources

Boardmaker Share:
http://www.boardmakershare.com/
Brainworks:
http://www.sensationalbrain.com/
CAST:
http://www.cast.org/udl/
Class Dojo:
https://www.classdojo.com/
Indiana Center for Accessible Materials (ICAM):
http://www.icam.k12.in.us/
Me Moves:
www.thinkingmoves.com
Model Me Kids:
http://www.modelmekids.com/
National Center on Universal Design for Learning:
http://www.udlcenter.org/
News to You:
https://www.n2y.com/news2you/
NIMAS:
http://aim.cast.org/learn/policy/federal/what_is_nimas
PATINS Universal Design Lesson Plans:
http://www.patinsproject.com/UDLLessons/udlteam.html
Paula Kluth:
http://www.paulakluth.com/category/autism/
Pinterest:
http://pinterest.com/theautismhelper/adapted-books-for-children-with-autism/
http://pinterest.com/search/pins/?q=differentiated%20instruction&rs=ac&len=8
Social Thinking Curriculum:
http://www.socialthinking.com/books-products
SticKids:
http://www.stickids.com/
SensoryTreat:
http://www.sensorytreat.com/
TEACCH:
http://www.teacch.com/
Teachers pay Teachers:
http://www.teacherspayteachers.com/
TeachTown:
http://web.teachtown.com/
Time Timer:
http://itunes.apple.com/us/app/time-timer/id332520417?mt=8
Visual Supports Module:

http://autismpdc.fpg.unc.edu/content/visual-supports
Visual Supports IRCA:
http://www.iidc.indiana.edu/index.php?pageId=3613

References

Busick, M., & Neitzel, J. (2009). *Self-management: Steps for implementation*. Chapel Hill, NC: National Professional Development Center on Autism Spectrum Disorders, Frank Porter Graham Child Development Institute, University of North Carolina.

Franzone, E. (2009). *Overview of task analysis*. Madison, WI: National Professional Development Center on Autism Spectrum Disorders, Waisman Center, University of Wisconsin.

Franzone, E., & Collet-Klingenberg, L. (2008). *Overview of video modeling*. Madison, WI: The National Professional Development Center on Autism Spectrum Disorders, Waisman Center, University of Wisconsin.

Gregory, G., & Chapman, C. (2013). *Differentiated instructional strategies: One size doesn't fit all* (3rd ed.). California: Corwin.

Hume, K. (2008). *Overview of visual supports*. Chapel Hill, NC: National Professional Development Center on Autism Spectrum Disorders, Frank Porter Graham Child Development Institute, The University of North Carolina.

Kluth, P., & Danaher, S. (2010). *From tutor scripts to talking sticks: 100 ways to differentiate instruction in K-12 inclusive classrooms*. Maryland: Brooks Publishing.

Premack, D. (1965). Reinforcement theory. In D. Levine (Ed.), *Nebraska symposium on motivation* (pp. 123–180). Lincoln: University of Nebraska Press.

Stansfeld, S. A., Berglund, B., Clark, C., Lopez Barrio, I., Fischer, P., Ohrstrom, E., et al. (2005). Aircraft and road traffic noise and children's cognition and health: Exposure-effect relationships. *The Lancet, 365*, 1942–1949.

Chapter 5
Collaborative Teaming: OT and SLP Co-treatment of Autism Spectrum Disorder

Kristi A. Jordan and Kristie Brown Lofland

A collaborative approach between speech-language pathologists (SLPs) and occupational therapists (OTs) is a highly effective treatment strategy, as the combination of the two therapeutic approaches allows therapists to address most of the core deficits and differences attributed to autism spectrum disorder (ASD). Language, communication, and social skills difficulties are one of the major core deficits listed in the diagnostic criteria of ASD (American Psychiatric Association 2013). Additional diagnostic criteria include sensory integration or processing differences, and sensory modulation differences, including hyper- and hypo-reactivity to sensory input. Individuals with these differences struggle to make sense of a world they cannot predict, organize, or respond to effectively.

The theory behind sensory integration is that it is the basis for all human behavior. As Dr. Ayres (1995) shared, sensory integration is "the process of organizing sensory inputs so that the brain produces a useful body response and also useful perceptions, emotions, and thoughts. Sensory integration sorts, orders, and eventually puts all of the individual sensory inputs together into a whole brain function. When the functions of the brain are whole and balanced, body movements are highly adaptive, learning is easy, and good behavior is a natural outcome."

Thus, if sensory input is not integrated purposefully and usefully, an individual is not able to respond consistently and in an adaptive way. This relates to the ability for a child to communicate successfully using verbal, nonverbal, and contextual information. An individual that cannot integrate sights, sounds, and other sensory inputs that compete with sight and sound is not able to respond to those inputs and produce an adaptive response, which would be the basis of communication.

Instead, individuals who do not take in or respond to sensory input adequately develop sensory sensitivities or sensory-seeking behaviors, stereotypical behaviors and vocalizations, abnormal body movements or awareness, and/or atypical speech sounds and patterns.

K.A. Jordan (✉) · K.B. Lofland
Indiana Resource Center for Autism, Indiana University, Bloomington, IN, USA
e-mail: krijorda@indiana.edu

K.B. Lofland
e-mail: klofland@indiana.edu

© Springer International Publishing Switzerland 2016
T.A. Cardon (ed.), *Technology and the Treatment of Children with Autism Spectrum Disorder*, Autism and Child Psychopathology Series,
DOI 10.1007/978-3-319-20872-5_5

In order to treat these differences, OTs and SLPs may find effective treatment lies in integrating sensory inputs into communication and evidence-based strategies, to allow the individual to maintain arousal, sustain optimal attention, react with expected emotions and affect, and engage purposefully in action as a response (Anzalone and Williamson 2001). These four A's are core to sensory integration theory regarding modulation (arousal, attention, affect, and action). Without these, successful interventions are very difficult to achieve.

Evaluation of oral-motor skills is often times overlooked when evaluating the treatment needs of students with ASD. Often times, programs that are trying to encourage verbal language development have not focused on the child's ability to process sensory information. The result is a system that cannot produce the movements needed for verbal imitation or to even produce a sound or a syllable. For example, if a child is hypersensitive to any tactile input in their mouth, they will not be able to produce a /d/ or /t/ sound that requires the tongue to make contact with the palate. Children with ASD are often unable to register and modulate sensory information in one or more of the sensory systems (Ayres 1979; Flanagan 2008). Not being able to register and modulate sensory information interferes with the development of oral-motor skills which in turn interferes with feeding skills, speech production, and communication.

Speech is considered to be vocal communication and is comprised of the sounds of language. Prior to the development of speech, communication begins at birth. Infants learn to communicate using their senses. They communicate through what they hear, see, touch, and feel, through their movement and interactions in their world.

Research has confirmed that infants show preferences for human faces over other stimuli, speech over other sounds within the environment, female voices over other voices, and the sound of their own mother's voice over other female's voices. They are able to use their sensory systems to facilitate and attend to what is most relevant and to inhibit, or ignore that which is less relevant. To communicate effectively, individuals must be able to exchange information.

Communication deficits are central to the diagnosis of ASD. However, the deficits are not only in language. The deficits exist more fundamentally in communication regardless of modality. A minority, approximately 20–30 % of children with ASD, do not develop spoken language as a primary means of communication. They also do not compensate for a lack of speech with gestures or other means of communication. Some individuals on the spectrum may be able to repeat sounds and speech, often referred to as echolalia, but may not be able to produce spontaneous and meaningful speech needed for communication. Other individuals are able to communicate, but need to be taught to use augmentative and alternative modes of communication to compensate for a lack of recognizable speech sounds. Often times, individuals will resort to the use of behaviors as communicative attempts.

Due to the integration of sensory and motor abilities into the development of speech and language skills, a natural connection between the occupational therapists and SLPs exists. SLPs and OTs have a common foundation of practice. Both disciplines are trained in allied health and medical health fields and share many prerequisite and core coursework. Both professions target daily functions and are trained in understanding anatomy, physiology, neurology, illnesses/disease processes, and medical management of disorders, in order to treat holistically. OT practice often prioritizes self-care, work, play, psychosocial function, motor skills, sensory integration, and related functional issues that impact participation in daily activities. SLPs prioritize functions of speech, communication, cognitive ability, and oral-motor skills that allow individuals to participate in daily activities.

The foundational connection between the two disciplines is the impact of the sensory and motor systems on daily life. If an individual cannot integrate sensory information within their environment, he/she will have difficulty with producing effective communication, speech, or motor response within that environment.

Both disciplines attempt to identify the etiology of presenting issues and diagnoses, and existing skill deficits or difficulties, and then use the process of task analysis to develop an effective treatment plan or therapeutic approach. Both professions are committed to facilitating the development of an individual's maximal functional potential to achieve independence and success in the skills required for daily life, such as self-care, mobility, and communication.

In particular in the pediatric population, there is often a developmental progression of skill acquisition. For example, in order to be successful at self-feeding, which is an activity of daily living that falls within the scope of an OT's practice, individuals must be able to use oral-motor skills to open and close their mouths and to use their mouths, tongues, and swallowing mechanisms to successfully eat, which falls within the scope of an SLP's practice. This overlap within one daily activity is an example of how there is a natural overlap of treating therapies, which results in a method of delivery often referred to as co-treatment. In a co-treatment session, multiple skills can be targeted cohesively with the same functional activity or goal.

Collaboration between SLP and OT allows practitioners to simultaneously target skills and treatment delivery to maximize effectiveness during treatment. If individuals are able to improve sensory processing, modulation, and motor response, they are more successful in developing a consistent and effective adaptive response to stimuli.

A collaborative session between disciplines, or co-treatment, allows both therapists to use their professional skills to prepare individuals for participation in a therapy session and address complimentary components of skill development. Successful collaboration allows the individuals to also generalize the skills taught within the therapy session into their home, classroom, or daily life. When in a collaborative or co-treatment session, the individual (or group) would be more likely to transition to therapy using sensory strategies, would then sit in an adapted seat or spot in the room versus traditional seating, and would incorporate multiple sensory and motor systems into learning.

Social Skills and Pragmatics

Individuals with ASD, social pragmatic communication disorders, and other related disabilities benefit from a co-treatment approach when addressing social skills. SLPs and OTs offer insight into both the assessment and treatment. Although any staff member can help with social skills instruction, SLPs and OTs are specifically trained to address psychosocial and social skills through their education in the subjects of psychology, group treatment, and social interaction skills. Social skills require individuals to have foundational cognitive and language skills. Additionally, sociocultural knowledge is necessary. OTs and SLPs can work with individuals on developing the necessary cognitive and linguistic skills required, including emotional processing, attention and working memory, executive function, and theory of mind. Individuals should be able to fluidly perform these skills within multiple settings.

Treatment Session Example

Treatment sessions are typically considered to be the time that an individual or group spends in direct treatment with the therapist providing services. Often it is believed that the session begins when the individual receiving therapy sits at the therapy desk or table and begins skill work. The effectiveness of therapy sessions may actually begin during transition from the classroom to the therapy room or from activity to activity, particularly in an inclusive educational setting. Social engagement and relatedness can be addressed from the moment the therapist or educator calls for the individual receiving therapy. The skills of timing and social interaction can continue to be addressed during the walk to the therapy setting or classroom. Daily living skills, following routines, and following directions can also be addressed in the context of preparing for therapy and during the transition. For example, if students are required to remove their shoes for therapy, the task of shoe-tying can be incorporated. This may be further aided by visual supports provided on a device, such as a task analysis app that provides step-by-step instructions with visual supports or through the use of previously taken digital photographs of each step of the required task being performed by the student. The student can simply access the photographs by touching the screen and swipe the photographs away, one at a time, in order to see the next step.

In fact, through the use of technology such as an iPad or tablet, a visual schedule can be used via applications or calendar functions. The visual support of a schedule allows the individual to improve their ability to transition more independently. Through use of technology for visual schedules, other organizing features and options become possible, such as pop-up task reminders with optional alarms. The same app or calendar program can also be used to create a sub-schedule or a task list. The sub-schedule can be presented to the individual to show him/her what will be happening in the therapy session. Communicating the basic principles of TEACCH (known as structured TEACCHing) by letting the individual know what work, how much work, when he/she is finished, and what is next promotes predictability. Structured TEACCHing practices reduce anxiety about the unknown aspects of a treatment session. In addition, a digital timer may also be used through the clock function on a device or through use of an application on the iPad or tablet. A timer can optionally be set for tasks to countdown to transition or to visually communicate how long each activity is expected to take. Timers are useful for individuals that do not become anxious by the visual reminder. Timers can also be set without being visually seen during a task if their use distracts or promotes anxiety in the individual.

Because of the collaborative nature of the treatment session with SLPs and OTs, skills targeted can include fine and gross motor, oral motor, sensory motor, articulation and language development, activities of daily living, writing and tool use, play/leisure, and social skill activities. The use of language during functional activities promotes generalization of skills and provides a framework of understanding to the activities being performed.

In a typical co-treatment session, the treating therapists will typically work with one to five individuals per session, depending on treatment goals. When individuals are seen for a co-treatment session, overlapping areas of concern or treatment priorities are grouped together according to related treatment goals or diagnoses.

For an example, when working with two individuals with ASD with speech articulation, language, and fine motor issues, a typical treatment session lesson plan may look as follows:

After checking a visual schedule app, photograph of the therapy room or area, or a calendar feature, the two individuals being seen for treatment transition to the therapy room or area. While walking to the therapy room, the same devices would be used for greetings or to visually support individuals by reminding them to greet one another. Through use of voice output, the individuals are able to greet adults or peers encountered during the transition. Each individual is given the support or prompt that is individually needed. If one requires only a visual support, then this is the extent of the prompt given. If the other individual needs voice output, technology allows that individual to successfully great peers and adults. Other individuals may simply need the visual reminder prior to transition. Some may require additional gestures, verbal, and/or visual prompts to participate.

Upon entering the therapy room, both individuals will be visually and verbally directed to the therapy room or area. Routines are built to allow individuals to predict what will happen and changes are incorporated systematically, through visual prompts and priming.

Depending on the treatment setting, OT may choose to begin the session by incorporating various low- and high-tech sensory and fine motor activities, such as fidget use, gross motor sensory activities, or use of therapy putty exercises to prepare their bodies for the session. After preparation, the individuals may then be seen separately by each therapist, with the therapists and individuals switching after a designated time or task.

The SLP will be using a variety of low- and high-tech options, such as an app that practices articulation skills, while the OT simultaneously works with the other individual using similar tools such as an iPad or tablet, but may be working on a different set of skills, such as fine or visual motor activities.

Social Benefits of Groups and/or Co-treatment

By working together on activities, individuals can then benefit from opportunities to develop social skills. Through use of photograph and video features on the devices used, video modeling can be used to demonstrate an activity and additional apps or activities can be used to deliver social skills instruction. Individuals are then afforded the opportunity to practice social skills and generalize skills previously being practiced, such as writing/speaking a story together, role playing a social skill, or through playing a game and learning concepts such as turn-taking or maintaining conversation. Following this activity, therapists may choose to allow individuals to choose an activity as reinforcement for completing the treatment activities assigned. This choice time should be incorporated in the visual schedule or sub-schedule/agenda for the session.

Reduce Materials

Use of technology allows the therapists to work on a variety of skills without having to switch out or manage a large amount of physical material. For example, the SLP can work on articulation skills that previously would have used flash cards, stampers, and work sheets and the OT is working on fine motor and visual motor tasks that would have required puzzles, pieces, worksheets, pencils, and crayons to be accessible. Through the use of a tablet or iPad, the same treatment objectives can be met and activities can be switched or adapted more readily. The OT can incorporate tools, such as a stylus to address handwriting skills.

Data Collection

Data collection is simplified with the use of multi-feature apps. The SLP and OT could choose to use the same app and writing prompt to then voice record the session with the individual and collect data on the student's responses during this session. This one activity completed on the app is saved to collect data on multiple treatment goals, related to the individual's plan. The OT can later review the student's writing sample through accessing the app or by taking a quick screenshot of the writing sample and emailing it or saving it to a digital file.

When each activity is completed, the individuals can continue to switch or may work together. Again, both the SLP and OT will be able to collect data related to their shared or independent goals and save examples of the individual's work samples.

Sensory Ideas for Co-treatment

Organization

The OT and SLP need toreate-organized treatment spaces that will help individuals to organize their brains, bodies, and sensory responses. An organized environment promotes a calm sensory response. Designated spaces should have clear visual boundaries to indicate what is to occur. Supplies and belongings should be organized in specific locations within designated spaces. Co-treating therapists should consider using structured work tasks and systems to organize work and activities. Use of visual supports during the session to prepare, inform, teach, and self-monitor will assist in self-management and comprehension.

Spaces

Co-treating therapists can create calm spaces within treatment areas, with soft materials, low light, and closed areas where individuals can take time to organize their systems when overwhelmed. They can also provide consultation to classroom teachers and building staff on how to incorporate this strategy building-wide. Within the treatment space, therapists can also provide opportunities for movement that organizes, such as rocking in a rocking chair or sitting on a therapy ball during treatment sessions. Co-treating therapists should pair movement with learning.

Modulation and Arousal

When planning activities in a therapy session, it is important to consider arousal level. Arousal level affects an individual's performance. If arousal level is too high, performance decreases due to inability to maintain attention and increased anxiety, among other factors. If arousal level is too low, performance decreases due to an inability to purposefully engage and sustain attention or motivation for a given task. To increase arousal, try incorporating alerting activities, such as standing during some activities, writing on a vertical surface, use of alternative seating, and through incorporating short movement breaks. Therapists could include transition walks (animal, robot, etc.) for younger students. To provide organizing input, have older students carry objects or "therapy bags" to the session. Include individuals in tasks, such as erasing a large dry erase board before the session. Oral motor and tactile input at the beginning of the session can also provide needed sensory input to organize and engage students. When an individual has optimal arousal, attention is sustained and a purposeful action, or response, is the result.

Sensory Defensiveness

For some individuals, sensory input can be distressing. It is a challenge for SLPs and OTs to address oral motor or fine motor issues when faced with sensory defensiveness, particularly tactile, oral, or auditory sensitivities. Individuals with tactile defensiveness may have difficulty tolerating touch, clothing textures, grooming, and self-care activities. Providing input that does not increase anxiety and opportunities for individuals to explore sensory input in a non-threatening way allows their systems to process and integrate the sensory experiences and produce an adapted and functional response.

For tactile and oral sensory de-sensitization, therapists should use caution in forcing any sensory input. It is important to respect that individual's personal space and to find a balance between being gentle and firm when approaching sensitivities. Distress or signs of fear and anxiety can reduce an individual's ability to respond and adapt. Therapists should use clinical skills and judgment in transitioning to more intense input and should recognize if an individual can or cannot tolerate given inputs. Use of inhibitory input, such as proprioceptive input, will allow therapists to address defensiveness. An example of this would be to use Lycra to provide deep pressure and to provide chew tubes, blowing activities, or chewy snacks throughout the day.

Oral and Verbal Praxis

When individuals have difficulties with oral praxis, they may have difficulty with tongue movements, lip control, sucking, swallowing, and eating. They may struggle with imitating oral movements. If they have differences with verbal praxis, they may struggle with articulation of speech and with planning and executing with conversation (sentences). Again, incorporating fun and interactive activities and games to improve ideation, awareness, and planning of oral-motor skills will allow therapists to address oral praxis within a therapy session. Include activities that require tongue, lip, cheek, and facial imitation and independently initiated movements.

Conclusion

Combining speech-language pathology and occupational therapy allows for an effective treatment approach for individuals with ASD. Collaborative treatment between OTs and SLPs that incorporates sensory strategies into evidence-based communication strategies allows therapists to impact modulation of sensory information and improve learning. If individuals adequately modulate and integrate sensory information, they are able to maintain arousal, sustain optimal attention, react with expected emotions and affect, and engage purposefully in communication as a response.

References

American Psychiatric Association. (2013). Diagnostic and statistical manual of mental disorders (5th ed.). Washington, DC.

Anzalone, M. E., & Williamson, G. (2001). *Sensory integration and self-regulation in infants and toddlers: Helping very young children interact with their environment.* Washington, DC: Zero to Three.

Ayres, J. A. (1995/1979). *Sensory integration and the child* (12th ed.). California: Western Psychological Services.

Flanagan, M. (2008). *Improving speech and eating skills in children with autism spectrum disorders—an oral-motor program for home and school.* Shawnee, Kansas: Autism Asperger Publishing Company.

Kranowitz, C. (1998). *The out-of-sync-child.* New York: Berkley Publishing Group.

Levels of the Ziggurat. http://texasautism.com/blog/levels/.

National Professional Development Center on Autism Spectrum Disorders. (2008). *Evidence based practices for children and youth with ASD.* Retrieved from http://autismpdc.fpg.unc.edu/content/briefs/.

Chapter 6
Supporting the Writing Skills of Individuals with Autism Spectrum Disorder Through Assistive Technologies

Amy Bixler Coffin, Brenda Smith Myles, Jan Rogers and Wendy Szakacs

The elements of written expression—handwriting, prewriting, writing, and writing conventions—require a set of complicated skills that go beyond the act of holding a pencil and putting words on paper. It includes the complex interaction among physical, cognitive, and sensory systems (Kushki et al. 2011). Most students with autism spectrum disorder (ASD) are likely to have difficulties with written expression which will impact their academic performance across subject matter areas (Griswold et al. 2002; Whitby and Mancil 2009). This paper highlights some of the challenges experience by writers with ASD as well as assistive technology supports that can positively impact (a) handwriting; (b) the prewriting process; (c) the writing process that includes drafting, editing, revising, and the final product; and (d) writing conventions that include spelling and grammar.

Characteristics of ASD that Impact Written Expression

ASD is associated with a high occurrence of motor difficulties (Gowan and Hamilton 2013) that impact the physical aspects of handwriting: postural control, motor control, motor memory, and motor planning (Fournier et al. 2010). Consistent with impairments in motor planning is a high prevalence of dyspraxia in individuals on the autism spectrum. Dyspraxia, the disruption in the way messages from the brain are communicated to the body, affects a person's ability to perform smooth, coordinated movements, those needed when performing fine motor skills

A.B. Coffin (✉) · B.S. Myles · J. Rogers · W. Szakacs
Ohio Center for Autism and Low Incidence, Columbus, OH, USA
e-mail: amy_bixler@ocali.org

B.S. Myles
e-mail: brenda_myles@me.com

J. Rogers
e-mail: jan_rogers@ocali.org

W. Szakacs
e-mail: wendy_szakacs@ocali.org

© Springer International Publishing Switzerland 2016   59
T.A. Cardon (ed.), *Technology and the Treatment of Children with Autism Spectrum Disorder*, Autism and Child Psychopathology Series,
DOI 10.1007/978-3-319-20872-5_6

such as handwriting. Further, ASD is also associated with differences in manual dexterity, muscle tone, and grip strength (Kushki et al. 2011).

When students struggle with handwriting, there can be unfavorable implications on writing assignments. Letter formation, size, alignment, spacing, and overall legibility are often compromised (Kushki et al. 2011; Myles et al. 2003). Consequently, academic participation and performance can be affected. Demonstration of what the student knows about a particular subject or the ability to express his/her thoughts or opinions on a topic can be jeopardized when hand-writing is compromised (Delano 2007). It takes great attention to write legibly, oftentimes interfering with the focus on the writing assignment itself and ultimately causing undue stress on the individual. In addition, handwriting challenges can hinder students from keeping up with the excessive amount of written work required in school, eventually having a negative impact on educational performance (Church et al. 2000).

Writing is highly dependent on executive function components, including planning, working memory, cognitive flexibility, and inhibition (Hill 2004). Individuals on the autism spectrum frequently struggle in the writing process and need support in the early development of their writing. Getting ready to write and preparing for the actual composition can be very challenging for them. Questions such as "Where do I begin? Where and how do I find information on the topic? How do I organize all of the information that I gather? and How do I stay focused on the assignment and complete it in the required timeline?" are frequently posed by writers, yet the answers to such questions do not come easily to individuals on the autism spectrum. For this reason, supports are needed to aid in the writing process (Dockrell et al. 2014).

In addition, characteristics associated with ASD, such as deficits in theory of mind (ToM), or the ability to consider another person's viewpoint; difficulty engaging in abstract and imaginative thinking; and weak central coherence, or the inability to see the "big picture" and instead focusing only on the details, can negatively impact a person's ability to successfully participate in the writing pro-cess (cf., Brown and Klein 2011; Fuentes et al. 2010). Furthermore, differences in language and communication skills as they relate to gathering and expressing thoughts in a cohesive fashion and then expressing them on paper can also jeop-ardize the writing process (Asaro-Saddler and Bak 2014).

Myriad research has shown that the brains of individuals with ASD operate differently than those without autism (cf., Anagnostou and Taylor 2011; Brambilla et al. 2003) and, consequently, there is an impact on written expression (Dockrell et al. 2014). The different parts of the brain do not communicate with one another in a manner similar to the brains of typically developing students. The ability to write involves an extreme amount of synchronization between the parts of the brain governing motor control, language skills, sensory feedback, and executive function (Boucher and Oehler 2013). When this does not occur, coordination of the skills needed for written expression is negatively influenced resulting in an interruption in the flow and planning of thoughts and their transformation into text (Asaro-Saddler and Saddler 2010). For example, if a student has language deficits, it may be difficult for her to generate ideas on paper. In addition, she may struggle with formulating sentences and/or paragraphs and organizing them in a way that makes sense to the reader. Simultaneously, the act of actually using a pencil may trigger anxiety due to motor challenges.

Handwriting Strategies

The act of being able to efficiently and effectively handwrite, as was mentioned previously, can be challenging for individuals with ASD. However, there are many different types of assistive technologies that can help to support difficulties with handwriting. It is extremely important to conduct an AT assessment that addresses the various components of handwriting so that appropriate assistive technology features can be selected based on the student's specific needs (Beigel 2000). It can also be helpful to adapt and support the actual process of handwriting by first looking at both the writing implements and the paper accommodations before looking for higher tech alternatives to handwriting, such as keyboarding and touch screen devices. Sometimes, the lower tech solutions can be implemented more easily and with minimal learning invested by the student (Alper and Raharinirina 2006). This section will present various AT features of writing supports because features matching is one of the most important and critical parts of the AT assessment process.

Sensory AT Feature Accommodations

Sensory challenges faced by individuals with ASD may be in the form of sensitivities or decreased responsiveness to sensory input (Myles et al. 2014). Both can create challenges in holding writing implements and executing strokes for handwriting. Tool features that may be useful for individuals who are sensory sensitive may include trying various sizes, shapes, textures, and types of writing utensils to see which are most sensory acceptable to the student. In addition to the actual writing implement, writing paper and surfaces can also impact students with sensory sensitivities (Fuentes et al. 2009). Consideration for the type, color, and texture of the paper used may be necessary. Some students may also have a sensory preference for the drag of the pencil or pen on the writing surface. Dry erase boards or gel pens offer a harder and smoother writing experience with less drag, whereas fine point pens and thicker papers may offer more resistance when writing. Finally, individuals with autism may also not only have tactile and kinesthetic sensitivities, but some also have visual sensitivities to the paper and text color (Ludlow et al. 2008). Color screens tests may be useful in determining which colors are more effective in supporting the writing needs for a specific student (Wizla 2012).

If a student is an emergent writer who has difficulty holding a writing implement due to sensory sensitivities, sometimes touch screen technologies offer an alternative to support the student's future use of writing tools (Pennington 2010). Often, a finger can be used to create letters/words/sentences that are displayed on the screen without the need to hold a writing implement, allowing the student to develop the kinesthetic feel of the letter formation without also dealing with the challenge of holding the utensil simultaneously. This may be done through built-in handwriting recognition within the touch screen device or through separate apps, particularly drawing apps. Because of the smaller size of most touch screens and the size of the strokes made by a finger, this is typically not a good solution for those who plan to generate a large amount of text. However, there are now styli that can be worn on the finger rather than held like a writing implement. These styli can be used to create a more localized touch by the finger resulting in a smaller stroke that may allow for more text entry than previously provided by finger strokes. Some apps, particularly those developed specifically for drawing, also allow the option to adjust the size of the mark created by the finger despite the actual size of the finger. However, generally speaking, the use of a finger to provide handwritten input on a touch screen is best used for students who are emergent drawers/writers to help facilitate the understanding that movements captured on paper have meaning and to further develop kinesthetic awareness of the formation of letters.

Students with decreased sensory responsiveness may benefit from a trial of weighted writing utensils, as well as those that provide more drag on the writing surface such as fine tip pens, soft pencil leads, and chalk. Writing surfaces and papers with texture and increased thickness may also provide additional resistance and input. Increasing the weight and resistance is sometime helpful in providing the additional sensory input the student needs (Myles et al. 2014). There is often a fairly wide variation in what each individual student finds as an acceptable writing utensil and paper based on sensory preferences and needs. Experimenting with a variety of utensils and papers with consideration for the above features could help to narrow down the choices.

Postural/Motor AT Feature Accommodations

Individual with ASD may demonstrate motor challenges that include poor body awareness, proximal stability, and generalized weakness. These challenges can directly impact handwriting output in terms of speed, quality, and endurance (Fournier et al. 2010). However, before the actual motor impact of writing is addressed, the student's general seating and positioning should be considered, as this also will impact handwriting success (Tomchek and Case-Smith 2009).

While seating and positioning assistive technology options will not be discussed in detail in this chapter, the reader should be aware of general guidelines for appropriate seating of all students. Desk and chair heights should be adjusted such that students are able to sit comfortably at the desk with the full surface of their feet firmly on the floor. They should also be able to rest elbows on the desk at a natural height for appropriate support and have adequate reach to engage in the activity of handwriting. Students with more significant weakness and low tone issues will likely need additional postural and seating supports beyond that which is provided with an appropriately sized standard classroom desk and chair. An occupational and/or physical therapist should assess these additional accommodations. It is important to address these issues before making other handwriting accommodations, and appropriate seating support often positively impacts handwriting performance without additional or with fewer accommodations.

Some individuals with ASD may demonstrate alternate grasp patterns of writing implements that may in part be related to sensory sensitivities, low muscle tone, and/or weakness. Pencil grips that offer visual cues for specific finger placement locations may be useful to encourage students who need help finding and developing a functional grasp pattern.

For students who have decreased strength and weakness as an underlying issue to handwriting challenges, large barrel writing utensils are sometimes helpful. Wearable writing implements that support the appropriate positioning and reduce the grasp needed to hold the writing implement may also be helpful. They may also benefit from writing surfaces that are smooth and offer little resistance of the writing implement on the writing surface such as dry erase boards (Tomchek and Case-Smith 2009).

Visual Motor at Feature Accommodations

Some individuals with autism may have underlying deficits in visual motor integration impacting their ability to execute letter and word formations including the appropriate sizing and spacing of letters. Specifically, macrographia, which is characterized by excessively large handwriting, is a common issue found in the handwriting of individuals with ASD (Johnson et al. 2013). These types of challenges may be supported by using specialized papers that have tactile and/or visual cues.

Papers that offer tactile cues often have one or more of the writing lines raised so students can feel the line with their writing implement when they bump up against it. These types of papers can be commercially purchased or they can also be made with puffy paints or liquid white glue by tracing over the lines on the paper and then allowing the paint/glue to dry before use. These papers can be helpful for guiding the student in appropriate letter and word sizing.

Specialty papers with visual cues can include many variations that provide visual cues for lines and spaces. Many times these papers can be used to support instruction in handwriting development, as well as provide ongoing visual supports for maintenance of developed skills. There are papers with different line/boundary types such as dashed lines, dotted lines, bold lines, and letter boxes. There are also papers with color-coding such that both lines and writing spaces may be color-coded. In addition, papers with pictures of supports on the lines delineate the top, middle, and lower lines for writing.

Writing Speed and Legibility AT Feature Accommodation

Despite efforts to accommodate sensory motor and visual motor needs with standard and alternative writing implements and papers, some students with autism may not be able to use those accommodations successfully for effective writing speed and legibility (Trewin and Arnott 2009). For those students keyboarding, touch screen technologies, scanning, and speech-to-text technologies may offer handwriting alternatives that still allow the students to generate written text independently but in a digital text format. Oftentimes, these solutions can also help to increase the overall legibility of the written product, as well as the speed at which the student is able to generate text.

The use of keyboarding as a successful alternative to handwriting for students with ASD has been noted in the research (Tomchek and Case-Smith 2009). Keyboarding can offer support for students who may have sensory motor or visual perceptual challenges that impact the production of handwritten output (Hellinckz et al. 2013). Keyboarding has been found to offer improved legibility and speed of written output for some students with ASD. There are many different types of keyboard options available. Oftentimes, students do very well with a standard keyboard attached to a desktop or laptop computer. There are also dedicated portable word processing devices such as the Forte and Fusion by Writer Learning. These types of devices offer an easy-to-use interface that includes features that support only the writing process. There are typically no additional features in the portable word processors that can create distractions for students, such as Internet access, games, programs, or apps. These devices are simple writing support systems only. Features that may be found on these types of devices include text-to-speech, word prediction, spelling check, and electronic writing rubrics. The screens typically display four-to-six lines of text at a time which can be a disadvantage for some students who need to see all content while composing. However, the text generated on these devices can be sent to a computer via Bluetooth and/or cable connection for final editing in a word processing document.

In addition to the standard keyboard, there are also many different types of specialized keyboards, such as keyboards with alternate key layouts (ABC, Dvorak, etc.), large and small footprint keyboards, color-coded keyboards, and programmable keyboards (Trewin and Arnott 2009). The alternate keyboard offers potential for some students with ASD who may need more intensive supports through the expanded keyboard. That type of keyboard offers features that may support motor challenges, such as the ability to create custom key layouts of various key sizes and spacing as well as adjustable touch sensitivity. Its greatest strength is in the custom content support it can provide for compositional writing.

Touch window or mobile devices such as the Google Chrome Book, Apple iPad, or smartphones when paired with specific writing apps or extensions offer features that have not been available in previous computer and keyboard technologies. Annotated note applications often offer features, such as the ability to take a picture of content and then draw, type, record, or handwrite to annotate the photographed information. This can help to reduce the quantity of handwriting required when taking notes either during lectures or when researching information for papers. Dedicated voice recording devices and apps are another way to reduce the need for handwriting. There are a number of apps that will allow recording of information, along with tagging for later retrieval. Devices, such as the LiveScribe Pen, are unique in that they allow a student the option of both taking typical handwritten notes in a special paper notebook and supplement those notes with a recording of a lecture. The benefit of this type of device as opposed to a standard digital recorder is that the recording actually attaches to the student's handwritten note, so the student can play back the recorded content that occurred when the handwritten note was taken. This could be useful for students who prefer to draw pictures or take cursory notes to represent content as well as students who fall behind in their note-taking due to slow handwriting speeds. These options are good for students who are gathering information, but do not expect to edit the information at a later date.

For those students who need to be able to reproduce hard copy text and then quickly use and edit the text at a later date, there are handheld scanners and apps that provide optimal character representation (OCR) technology to convert the scanned or photographed text (Puckett 2011). Dedicated handheld scanning devices can be used to reproduce text from hard copy sources so the information can be quoted or paraphrased for papers and reports at a later time. These devices allow for scanning of content in a specific location or several locations on a single page of text when the full text on the page of the document is not needed. Apps generally provide a way to photograph a full page of text at one time and then convert the hard copy text to editable digital text. Again this reduces the student's need to handwrite all information and increases their speed in gathering needed information.

Finally, speech-to-text provides yet another option to reduce or replace hand-writing, as well as typing (Puckett 2011). Speech-to-text, voice recognition, or automatic speech recognition are all often used synonymously to refer to the act of speaking into a computer or touch screen device, resulting in the device recognizing and converting the spoken words into editable digital text. The generated text can occur in word processing documents, text messages, e-mails, and most fields that can accept typed text. Many smartphones and touch screen technologies now provide speech-to-text within their platforms, as well as newer computer operating systems. There are also computer programs and applications that are specifically designed for generating speech-to-text. These types of programs can provide a higher degree of accuracy in interpreting an individual's speech patterns for the production of typed text as opposed to those found in various system platforms; however, there is generally a training period and a need to correct errors to keep the accuracy of the speech-to-text system working effectively. There are many considerations to using speech-to-text systems some of which include the noise in the immediate environment, the noise the user will make in the environment using the system, and the person's speech intelligibility, just to name a few. A more in-depth look at the various considerations for effective use of speech-to-text can be found at http://www.atinternetmodules.org/mod_intro.php?mod_id=96.

In summary, there are many features of AT and general technology tools that may help to support the handwriting needs of a student with ASD; however, in order to determine which tools may be most useful, it is necessary to assess learner needs, environments, and specific handwriting tasks to determine the most appropriate features and, ultimately, the specific tools that contain the needed features. It is recommended that accommodations to typical writing implements and papers be considered first and if the student is not able to adequately perform needed writing tasks with those types of tools that handwriting replacement tools be considered, such as those that provide digital text production capabilities through keyboarding, scanning, or voice recognition.

Prewriting Strategies

The beginning stage of the writing process is prewriting which includes (a) understanding an assigned topic or choosing a topic, (b) identifying main ideas, (c) finding supporting information for the main idea, and (d) organizing the information. Individuals with ASD may need additional direct instruction, a further breakdown of the assignment parts, and specific strategies or tools in order to complete prewriting successfully.

As a student begins the prewriting stage, a topic is either assigned or chosen. If at all possible, including a student's special interest area as a topic or a facet of a topic can be a motivational tool (Winter-Messiers 2007). A student would first research the assigned topic or possible topics through a variety of search engines and gather the initial information. For a student with ASD, this first step of prewriting can be overwhelming without further direction and supports. Once the student has decided on a topic, the next step is to support the topic with main ideas and supporting facts for each main idea. Then, all of this information needs to be organized in readiness for the actual writing. There are many smaller actions within each of these steps that can impact the quality of the project. As discussed earlier, a student with ASD may be challenged with how to begin any one of these steps, with where to find the information and decide what is applicable to the topic, and with figuring out a schedule of what to do and when to do it. There are some strategies and tools to help students with ASD approach prewriting in a more successful manner.

A first question for the student with ASD may be, "Where do I find the information and research?" At this point, a list of related books and a list of search engines could be helpful. Some search engines, such as Google Custom Search, iPL2, Sweet Search, or KidsClick, can be content specific and kid friendly. One site, Twurdy, displays search results at a needed readability level. Some students with ASD may need more specific search parameters through an individualized list of pages to visit or a form to fill in with a limited amount of information and a teacher check in for guidance before continuing.

When the student is researching a possible topic, mapping or graphic organizers (GO) can help make this more visual as compared to a listing of text representing the facts or thoughts (Twyman and Tindal 2006). Mapping or GO tools can be used at all age levels and individualized to meet the needs of a student. For instance, younger children may use the Five Fingered Planner that has students drawing or writing on the outline of a hand. The palm of the hand contains the topic, each finger has one detail, and the thumb relates a feeling the child has about the topic. An older child may use a bubbled outline in which each area contains a point and supporting details. Some students may use a virtual mapping or GO tool, such as Mindmeister, Text 2 Mind Map, or Essay Map, to organize the information found in the research stage.

Once the research information is gathered, the student will identify the main ideas and supporting details. Again, the use of mapping or GO can help make this step visual for the student with ASD. Direct instruction or a student–teacher conference may be necessary to help the learner narrow a topic and identify main ideas and supporting details.

The final step of prewriting is to organize the information sequentially. This may be supported through use of a template that uses a sequence of order, such as first, next, and then. Again, modeling how to organize the information using a variety of paper/pencil or virtual templates can support the learner's skills development. Again, direct instruction may be necessary for some individuals on the spectrum.

To address the executive function needs that arise during the writing process, particularly those related to organization (Nyden et al. 1999), there are several tools that can be used. If a student is challenged to complete a project with the basic instructions usually presented, then written or pictorial step-by-step instructions may be needed. Start with a task analysis of the project and then decide how far the student needs this project to be broken down to reach the highest level of success. Having a text, pictorial or virtual checklist of steps needed to complete the prewriting process can assist the student with ASD in completing all parts of the assignment (Myles and Rogers 2014).

Another executive function skill that may be challenging for those on the spectrum is time management (Mintz et al. 2012). Each step of the prewriting process needs to be completed within a given time period. Building in checkpoints or reminders can help the student with ASD move through the process in a timely manner. Reminders can be a star with text stating "Check-in with teacher today" or can be a virtual alarm that is available on iCal, CalAlarm, or Google Calendar. Apps, such as Countdown Calendar, show how many days are left until something is due. Similarly, iHomework allows a project to be chunked into smaller parts and has a reminder for each segment.

Keep in mind, there are many tools and supports that can be put in place for a student with ASD, but usage of the tools must be taught through direct instruction and monitored as the student begins to implement them.

Strategies to Support Writing Conventions

Writing conventions are the rules of spelling and grammar needed by the student to technically perform the act of writing. As previously discussed, many students with ASD struggle with the conventions of writing for a number of reasons. Handwriting challenges might be one explanation for these difficulties as they may compromise the cognitive resources needed for writing in general including writing conventions (Hellinckx et al. 2013). In addition, deficits in working memory may make it challenging to consider and operationalize all aspects of the writing process simultaneously (Brenner et al. 2015). Finally, language deficits may impact not only pragmatics, but may have a more significant influence in terms of the production and understanding of grammatically correct content (Dockrell et al. 2014). Assistive technologies can support these various areas of writing challenges that are often experienced by students with ASD. As has been mentioned previously, assessment of need is necessary for the best selection of technology supports with consideration for the student's needs, environments, and tasks. The SETT framework (Zabala 2005) can help provide teams with a framework for discussing specific technology supports needed by the student.

Spelling AT Feature Accommodations

Historically spelling support occurred when students used a dictionary to look up words. For students to be successful in this, they needed some fairly effective encoding skills to actually locate the word in the dictionary to check the spelling. They also needed to be able to focus long enough to (a) complete the task by sorting through a large number of options, (b) locate the correct response, and (c) transfer the information from the source to their work. Thus, multiple steps were needed that contained many opportunities for failure along the way. It was not infrequent to hear teachers and students alike say, "How can I find the correct spelling of a word in the dictionary if I don't know how to spell the word?"

The advent of the electronic handheld spell-checker seemed to help some of the problems associated with standard dictionary lookups for spelling assistance. Electronic spell-checkers are handheld dedicated devices. That is, they do essentially nothing more than provide spelling support. They can provide this assistance to individuals who still wish to generate handwritten work, but need more guidance than offered through a standard dictionary. While a student still needs to enter the word they wish to know how to spell, they do not need the spelling accuracy required by a standard dictionary. Electronic spell-checkers are often able to phonetically search using common spelling errors and offer several choices of best guesses of the student's targeted word. Because they are electronic, some are also able to speak the word options and definitions of the words generated so the student can ensure it is the word they intended to spell. There are also apps that can now perform the same types of functions as electronic handheld spell-checkers. The advantage to a spell-checker app is that they are often loaded on smartphones and are readily available to the person in any environment, so carrying a secondary dedicated device is not needed.

If more spelling support is needed by the student or if the student is generating written work through electronic means, electronic spell-checkers that are embedded in computer operating systems or standard word processors may be useful. These typically provide a basic level of spelling support and often include a visual cue when a word has been misspelled. Sometimes, these systems offer in-line spelling correction choices, but most require that a student activates spell check when the document is completed that alerts the system to search and find spelling errors and offer correction choices.

More sophisticated reading and writing support software specifically designed for students with disabilities, such as Kurzweil, Read and Write Gold, WYNN, and Solo, offer the greatest degree of spelling support. These feature-rich programs provide many different choices of spelling assistance in addition to other built-in reading and writing support tools. Several of the developers of these programs have also recently developed apps that provide some of the same spelling features as the full software programs. Spelling support in these tools may include different types of visual cues for misspelled words, such as highlighting, underlining, and flashing words. They may also include added auditory supports, such as playing a sound when a word is misspelled. All of these spell check features can occur in real time or can be set so that spell check can be manually activated by the student when desired. For many students with ASD, hyper-focusing on details, such as the identified misspelled words during real-time spell check, can create difficulties for the student in generating fluid thoughts during the writing process. Turning off the spell check and the constant reminders of misspelled words may reduce this difficulty. Once the student is finished getting her thoughts on paper, then the spell check can be activated with the appropriate visual and auditory cues.

All of the previously mentioned reading and writing programs have some type of phonetic spell check. Generally, this allows the spell check to effectively return spelling suggestions even when the student has provided phonetically misspelled words, words without vowels or has mirror letter errors. Because the spell check occurs within the written document, it can also use the context of the written work to better predict the word the student is attempting to spell, adding to the accuracy of the spell check for those students with significant challenges in spelling. Returned spelling suggestions are also generally provided with definitions in these programs. This can be extremely helpful to students with ASD who often struggle with the understanding of word meanings (Henderson et al. 2015). This can help to build vocabulary and ensure the correct replacement word is selected for the misspelled word. In addition, all of these programs provide a text-to-speech feature in the spell check so word choices can be spoken aloud to the student.

Many reading and writing programs also offer a word prediction feature that can support students with significant spelling challenges (Kagohara et al. 2012). This feature allows for the prediction of words as a student keyboards. It is not necessary for the student to type the entire word to see potential word choices. The word prediction found in these programs is different than the word completion that is found in smartphone technologies. The word prediction found in the reading and writing programs relies on the context of the written output and learns from the writer's writing style. It also includes many methods to generate word choices that enhance accuracy.

Word prediction can provide additional support for students with the most complex spelling challenges beyond traditional spell check in that it is interactive and generates word choices in real time. This real-time, automatic generation of words can also support students who have limited writing vocabularies and are not sure how to grammatically use words within sentences. In addition, it allows the student to see potential words that might be considered for the development of a sentence. Oftentimes, word prediction in these programs can be populated with custom word dictionaries so that words generated in the word prediction are specific to the student's writing topic. For example, if a student is writing about the Transcontinental Railway, he may see words in the word prediction such as transcontinental, railroad, Pacific, construction, continents, regions, and California with greater frequency. Again, this can be useful for students with ASD who may struggle with the understanding and use of vocabulary (Henderson et al. 2015). Some programs with word prediction, such as Intellitools Classroom Suite, also provide the option to activate pictures supports to accompany some words in the generated word prediction lists. For those students with emergent reading and writing skills who need that level of support, this is a great additional feature.

Grammar AT Feature Accommodations

If a student struggles using appropriate grammar during writing activities, technology supports are available through traditional word processing programs and with a greater degree of support through the specialized reading and writing programs mentioned previously in the spelling section. Most word processing programs have a grammar checker embedded in the program. Those can offer support for more advanced student writing; however, if students have more complex needs, those may be better met by using programs that are designed specifically for students with disabilities (Alliano et al. 2012).

The reading and writing programs mentioned previously have a number of "checker" features that can be launched when a student has completed the writing process. There are verb, confusable word (homonym), and general grammar checkers. The verb checker will look for conflicts in verb tense and recommend a more appropriate choice. The confusable word or homophone checker will search for words such as to, too, and two and assess if they have been used properly in the sentence. Recommendations are then offered along with the dictionary meaning so the student can determine which of the homophones are the correct word selection. Grammar checkers assess word order and appropriate punctuation and make suggestions for changes to improve the overall grammatical quality of the student's writing.

Finally, for students who are at emergent writing levels and need a great deal of support in producing writing with appropriate grammar, there are programs such as Intellitools Classroom Suite and Clicker that can be custom–designed to provide students with writing grids or toolbars. These custom writing grids or toolbars can be color-coded for easy identification of parts of speech, or they can be set so students have forced selections in appropriate grammatical order. With forced selection, only certain words are made available at a given time. The words, except those that are grammatically appropriate, may either be grayed out indicating they are not available for selection or they may not be visible until a selection is made from those that are available.

Summary

In summary, there are many tools available for students with ASD to support challenges in writing conventions. The tools can offer a minimal amount of support or can provide supports for students with the most complex challenges. Utilizing an assessment process can help to determine the appropriate amount of support needed by the student to support grammar and spelling difficulties and thus helping to identify the needed technology features.

References

Alliano, A., Herriger, K., Koutsoftas, A. D., & Bartolotta, T. E. (2012). A review of 21 iPad applications for augmentative and alternative communication purposes. *Perspectives on Augmentative and Alternative Communication, 21*, 60–71.

Alper, S., & Raharinirina, S. (2006). Assistive technology for individuals with disabilities: A review and synthesis of the literature. *Journal of Special Education Technology, 21*, 47–64.

Anagnostou, E., & Taylor, M. J. (2011). Review of neuroimaging in autism spectrum disorders: What have we learned and where we go from here. *Molecular Autism, 2*(4), 1–9.

Asaro-Saddler, K., & Bak, N. (2014). Persuasive writing and self-regulation training for writers with autism spectrum disorders. *Journal of Special Education, 48*, 92–105.

Asaro-Saddler, K., & Saddler, B. (2010). Planning instruction and self-regulation training: Effects on writers with autism spectrum disorders. *Exceptional Children, 77*, 107–124.

Beigel, A. R. (2000). Assistive technology assessment: More than the device. *Intervention in School and Clinic, 35*, 237–243.

Boucher, C., & Oehler, B. (2013). I hate to write: Tips for helping students with autism spectrum and related disorders increase achievement, meet academic standards, and become happy, successful writers. Shawnee Mission, KS: AAPC Publishing.

Brambilla, P., Hardan, A., Ucelli di Nemi, S., Perez, J., Soares, J. C., & Barale, F. (2003). Brain anatomy and development in autism: Review of structural MRI studies. *Brain Research Bulletin, 61*, 557–569.

Brenner, L. A., Shih, V. H., Colich, N. L., Sugar, C. A., Bearden, C. E., & Dapretto, M. (2015). Time reproduction performance is associated with age and working memory in high-functioning youth with autism spectrum disorder. *Autism Research, 8*, 29–37.

Brown, H. M., & Klein, P. D. (2011). Writing, Asperger syndrome, and theory of mind. *Journal of Autism and Developmental Disorders, 41*, 1464–1474.

Church, C., Alisanski, S., & Amanullah, S. (2000). The social, behavioral, and academic experiences of children with Asperger syndrome. *Focus on Autism and Other Developmental Disorders, 15*, 12–20.

Delano, (2007). Improving written language performance of adolescents with Asperger syndrome. *Journal of Applied Behavior Analysis, 40*, 345–351.

Dockrell, J. E., Ricketts, J., Charman, T., & Lindsay, G. (2014). Exploring writing products in students with language impairments and autism spectrum disorders. *Learning and Instruction, 32*, 81–90.

Fournier, K. A., Hass, C. J., Naik, S. K., Lodha, N., & Cauraugh, J. H. (2010). Motor coordination in autism spectrum disorders: A synthesis and meta-analysis. *Journal of Autism and Developmental Disorders, 40*, 1227–1240.

Fuentes, C. T., Mostofsky, S. H., & Bastian, A. J. (2009). Children with autism show specific handwriting impairments. *Neurology, 73*, 1532–1537.

Gowan, E., & Hamilton, A. (2013). Motor abilities in autism: A review of using a computational context. *Journal of Autism and Developmental Disorders, 43*(2), 323–344.

Griswold, D. E., Barnhill, G. P., Myles, B. S., Hagiwara, T., & Simpson, R. L. (2002). Asperger syndrome and academic achievement. *Focus on Autism and Other Developmental Disabilities, 17*(2), 94–102.

Hellinckx, T., Roeyers, H., & Van Waelvelde, H. (2013). Predictors of handwriting in children with autism spectrum disorder. *Research in Autism Spectrum Disorders, 7*, 176–186.

Henderson, L. M., Clarke, P. J., & Snowling, M. J. (2015). Accessing and selecting word meaning in autism spectrum disorder. *The Journal of Child Psychology and Psychiatry, 52*, 964–973.

Hill, E. L. (2004). Executive dysfunction in autism. *Trends in Cognitive Sciences, 8*(1), 26–32.

Johnson, B. P., Philips, J. G., Papadopoulos, N., Fielding, J., Tonge, B., & Rinehart, N. J. (2013). Understanding macrographia in children with autism spectrum disorders. *Research in Developmental Disabilities, 34*, 2917–2926.

Kagohara, D. M., Sigafoos, J. S., Achmadi, D., O'Reilly, M., & Lancioni, G. (2012). Teaching children with autism spectrum disorders to check the spelling of words. *Research in Autism Spectrum Disorders, 6*, 304–310.

Kushki, A., Chau, T., & Anagnostou, E. (2011). Handwriting difficulties in children with autism spectrum disorders: A scoping review. *Journal of Autism and Developmental Disorders, 41*, 1706–1716.

Ludlow, A. K., Wilkins, A. J., & Heaton, P. (2008). Colored overlays enhance visual perceptual performance in children with autism spectrum disorders. *Research in Autism Spectrum Disorders, 2*, 498–515.

Mintz, J., Branch, C., March, C., & Lerman, S. (2012). Key factors mediating the use of a mobile technology tool designed to develop social and life skills in children with autism spectrum disorders. *Computers & Education, 58*, 53–62.

Myles, B. S., Huggins, A., Rome-Lake, M., Hagiwara, T., Barnhill, G. P., & Griswold, D. E. (2003). Written language profile of children and youth with Asperger syndrome: From research to practice. *Education and Training in Developmental Disabilities*, 362–369.

Myles, B. S., Mahler, K., & Robbins, L. A. (2014). *Sensory issues and high functioning autism spectrum and related disorders: Practical solutions for making sense of the world*. Shawnee Mission, KS: AAPC Publishing.

Myles, B. S., & Rogers, J. (2014). Addressing executive function using assistive technology to increase access to the 21st Century Skills. In N. R. Stilton (Ed.), *Innovative technologies to benefit children on the autism spectrum* (pp. 20–34). Hershey, PA: IGI Global.

Nydén, A., Gillberg, C., Hjelmquist, E., & Heiman, M. (1999). Executive function/attention deficits in boys with Asperger syndrome, attention disorder and reading/writing disorder. *Autism, 3*, 213–228.

Pennington, R. C. (2010). Computer-assisted instruction for teaching academic skills to students with autism spectrum disorders: A review of literature. *Focus on Autism and Other Developmental Disabilities, 25*, 239–248.

Puckett, K. (2011). Technology applications for students with disabilities: tools to access curriculum content. In T. Bastiaens & M. Ebner (Eds.), *Proceedings of world conference on educational media and technology 2011* (pp. 3186–3191). Association for the Advancement of Computing in Education (AACE).

Tomchek, S. D., & Case-Smith, J. (2009). *Occupational therapy practice guidelines for children and adolescents with autism.* Bethesda, MD: AOTA Press.

Trewin, S., & Arnott, J. (2009). Text entry when movement is impaired. In I. Scott MacKenzie and K. Tahaka-Ishii (Eds.), *Text entry systems: Mobility, accessibility, and universality* (pp. 289–204). London, England: Morgan Kaufmann.

Twyman, T., & Tindal, G. (2006). Using a computer-adapted, conceptually based history text to increase comprehension and problem-solving skills of students with disabilities. *Journal of Special Education Technology, 21*, 5–16.

White, P. J. S., & Mancil, G. R. (2009). Academic achievement profiles of children with high functioning autism and Asperger syndrome: A review of the literature. *Education and Training in Developmental Disabilities, 44*, 551–560.

Winter-Messiers, M. A. (2007). From tarantulas to toilet brushes: Understanding the special areas of children and youth with Asperger syndrome. *Remedial and Special Education, 28*, 140–152.

Wizla, P. (2012, December 26). 10 Apps to help you tame your monitory at night. Retrieved January 10, 2015 from http://mac.appstorm.net/roundups/utilities-roundups/10-apps-to-help-you-tame-your-monitor-at-night/.

Zabala, J. S. (2005). Ready, SETT, go! Getting started with the SETT framework. *Closing the Gap, 23*(6), 1–3.

Chapter 7
Using Visual Organizers and Technology: Supporting Executive Function, Abstract Language Comprehension, and Social Learning

Ryan O. Kellems, Terisa P. Gabrielsen and Caroline Williams

Executive Function

Individuals with ASD frequently encounter challenges in the areas of attention, memory, and information processing due to impaired executive function skills. Executive functioning deficits commonly found with ASD include problems with planning, trouble with future-oriented thinking, challenges with organizing information, and difficulty with managing multiple tasks and with abstract problem solving (Coyne and Rood 2011; Hill and Bird 2006). These deficits fall under the traditional domain of executive function: planning, organization, time management, working memory, and metacognition (Dawson and Guare 2010).

Importance of Executive Function in the Classroom

Educational tasks in classroom environments require age-appropriate executive functioning for academic success (Coyne and Rood 2011). If executive function is delayed or impaired, as is the case in ASD, additional supports are needed for students to be successful. Individuals with ASD have been shown to have lower performance in tasks that require cognitive fluency, planning, goal setting, and shifting attention (Hill and Bird 2006; Kleinhans et al. 2005). Technology-enhanced visual strategies can be used to support individuals with ASD in classroom environments. These visual strategies require the student to plan and manage time

R.O. Kellems (✉) · T.P. Gabrielsen · C. Williams
Brigham Young University, Provo, UT, USA
e-mail: rkellems@byu.edu

T.P. Gabrielsen
e-mail: Terisa_Gabrielsen@byu.edu

© Springer International Publishing Switzerland 2016
T.A. Cardon (ed.), *Technology and the Treatment of Children with Autism Spectrum Disorder*, Autism and Child Psychopathology Series,
DOI 10.1007/978-3-319-20872-5_7

appropriately, set goals and subgoals for self-monitoring, and shift attention and cognition between multiple tasks. When strategies to support or ameliorate executive function deficits are employed by teachers, students with ASD have improved access to the curriculum (McKeon et al. 2013). Techniques for using technology-enhanced visual strategies to support both academic success and executive function are discussed in the next section.

Using Visual Strengths to Support Academic Success

Research has shown that many individuals with ASD have strengths in perceiving visual information (Roser et al. 2014); people with ASD learn and retain information when it is presented using visual supports (National Professional Development Center n.d.). Bryan and Gast (2000) hypothesized that young adults with ASD respond best to visual learning because they sometimes have difficulty comprehending and paying attention to auditory stimuli. When a student with ASD is struggling with educational tasks, the addition of visual supports to traditional instruction can help the student access information more efficiently (Hodgdon 2011).

Research supports the effectiveness of using visual supports for students with ASD. Kluth and Darmondy-Latham (2003) found that visually based instruction (i.e., Venn diagrams, graphic organizers, and flowcharts) when combined with verbal instructions was effective teaching strategies. Some individuals with ASD have difficulty seeing the whole picture (gestalt), and instead focus on details, sometimes at a superior level (Dakin and Frith 2005). These characteristics can be used, along with visual supports, to help a learner with ASD to succeed in difficult tasks, such as abstract concept comprehension and critical thinking.

Using Technology to Support Visual Learning Strengths

Advances in technology and affordability of devices for production of visually based interventions, such as video modeling and activity schedules, have made it easier than ever to provide visual supports in the classroom. For example, it is now possible to load multiple intervention videos and other applications onto a small device that can easily be carried around and used throughout the day, regardless of the setting. Students interact daily with socially acceptable, sophisticated devices that can deliver visually based instruction and reminders while integrating some unique interactive features. Students of all ages, including preschool students, commonly use handheld electronic devices such as iPods, iPads, tablets, cell phones, and computers for entertainment. Most students should be able to use one of these devices to easily incorporate watching a video modeling intervention, referring to a checklist, or consulting a visual map, and will be able to do so in a variety of different settings.

Electronic devices and technology are certainly attractive to individuals with ASD (Mineo et al. 2009) and have been shown to increase skill levels (King et al. 2014). Electronic devices can store large amounts of information, are portable, shareable, and easily updated. These devices provide flexibility—individuals can access interventions at home, at school, and in the community. Combining evidence-based interventions with technological strategies that have been shown to be attractive, effective methods of increasing skills in individuals with autism is the focus of the remainder of this chapter.

Supporting Academics Through Technology

Common Core State Standards (CCSS)

To date, 43 states, the District of Columbia, and four territories have adopted the Common Core State Standards (CCSS) (2014, retrieved from http://www.corestandards.org/about-the-standards). The CCSS are standards that have been developed for mathematics and English language arts. The CCSS now guide the general education assessments and curriculum for those two subjects. The standards are also being applied to courses other than math and English language arts. In states where CCSS have not been adopted, the state has a set of learning standards for each content area and grade level. These state standards can be used the same way CCSS are used.

In order for some students with ASD to meet the rigorous grade-level standards, adaptations to the general education instruction may be necessary. One adaptation that can easily be made is increased use of visually based instructional strategies when teaching CCSS-related content.

Literacy

In the Common Core for grades 9–10, students are expected to understand grade-level science textbooks and comprehend the terms in order to compare them to other scientific terms (CCSS.ELA-LITERACY.RST.9-10.5). This requirement emphasizes how crucial vocabulary knowledge is in classroom learning. Teachers can use computers to type up and post vocabulary around the room. Students can also use computers to create their own sentences using the vocabulary words (Broun 2004). There are also numerous Web sites available for students to explore. For example, quizlet.com allows the students to create their own vocabulary flash cards and monitor their progress. They can even compare their progress with others in the class. Another example is studyblue.com. Students can create their own vocabulary cards and use the Web site's library to add images to their cards.

Different apps are also available on the iPad and the iPhone. "Flashcards+" makes creating flash cards easy by allowing learners to create different categories, depending on which class they are working on. It also fosters vocabulary learning by allowing the student to access thousands of vocabulary cards that already exist.

As mentioned before, a deficit in executive functioning can impair an individual's ability to memorize pieces of information as a learning strategy (Coyne and Rood 2011). This may be true even if the individual has tremendous capacity for memorization of movie scripts or facts and figures. For this reason, students with autism cannot rely on memorization to master vocabulary terms. Memorization cannot help them apply the words to larger contexts or in comprehension strategies Jitendra et al. (2004). In order to comprehend, they need to establish relationships between words and apply them to different forms of text (Baumann and Kameenui 1991).

The Common Core's strong reliance on vocabulary makes learning difficult for those on the autism spectrum (Scruggs et al. 2013). The ability to create contextual relationships among different words in order to comprehend a passage is not a strength for those on the spectrum and puts them at a greater disadvantage.

To combat this, visual vocabulary can be used to help students with disabilities master new words. The words are printed and put up in the classroom for the student to see. In a vocabulary instruction method developed by Oelwein (1995), students with Down syndrome and other developmental delays were better able to learn the vocabulary through visualization and were then able to create sentences using the words.

Supporting Executive Function Through Technology

Visual Schedules

Visual schedules aid students with challenges related to autism spectrum disorders improve executive functioning and independence (National Autism Center 2009). Visual activity schedules, produced in a variety of ways, can be used to help individuals with ASD complete various tasks, understand what is required of them in a project, and help them learn daily routines. By providing the sequential steps in an accessible way, an individual can be successful and independent in completing a task that is not yet automatic or memorized, even if that task is part of a daily routine.

Behaviorally, visual schedules are a great tool to help reduce anxiety and disruptive behavior (Davies 2008). The schedule lessens anxiety that individuals with ASD may have about what is supposed to happen next. Reduced anxiety will likely alleviate challenging behaviors which leads to more learning time in the classroom. The process of completing each step, "checking it off," and then moving on to the next step helps the learner stay on task and engaged. Knowing what the next steps are, when the task is finished, and if there are any planned breaks in the schedule increases predictability (Banda et al. 2009).

Visual schedules can also be helpful in academic contexts. Specifically in history classes, visual schedules could be used to create timelines. The History Common Core standard for ninth grade asks the student to understand how different events impact the events that follow (CCSS.ELA-LITERACY.RH.9-10.3). Timelines can help learners organize the events in the proper order to better understand cause and effect. Web sites such as dipity.com can help students create their own timeline of different historic events. Not only are they involved in making the timelines, but the students can print them out and use them as a reference.

There are many resources that are available to create visual schedules. Different software can allow a teacher to import or choose images from a bank of pictures to create different sequences. Images can be printed, as in the past, but can also be used on computers and iPads.

Fortunately, there are numerous apps for the iPad and iPhone, smartphones, computers, and tablets that allow users to plan out their days (Table 7.1). Several apps allow users to create daily routine schedules or homework schedules. Other apps outline and break down various behavioral routines. This can be very beneficial for different procedures, such as transitioning between classes. Photographs or images can be used to represent the different tasks, and if video is the best modality for an individual to learn from, a video of each step in the task can be created, with built in pauses between steps to allow the individual to follow along.

Visual/Graphic Organizers

Visual organizers also have several academic support uses. A primary purpose may be to show a learner how different information is connected (Fisher and Schumaker 1995). Connections can be made in science as students use cause-and-effect, process-and-sequence, and compare-and-contrast graphic organizers (Grabe and Jiang 2007). Concepts that might be too abstract for individuals on the spectrum, such as the process of photosynthesis, can be made more concrete as the concept is broken down into steps in a process and sequence organizer. Graphic organizers can also help with comprehension as they activate a learner's prior knowledge and compare it to what is being taught (Kim et al. 2004).

In teaching literature, graphic organizers and story maps are viable tools to help those with ASD recognize different parts of the story (Stringfield et al. 2011). The Common Core requires that students in the sixth grade understand how different events and people contribute to the various dimensions of a story. Maps help learners fulfill this objective by allowing them to actively search for and fill out the various sections of the map, including setting, characters, and plot (CCSS. ELA-LITERACY.RL.6.5). Grasping the sequence of a story allows the learner to undertake the literature that has longer and more intricate story lines (Gately 2008).

Table 7.1 Technology resources for visual supports

Resource	Description/app
	Web site
Communication and time management aids	Variety of aids and technology for improving communication skills and executive function, including Boardmaker™ interactive applications
	www.mayer-johnson.com
Checklists for academic projects	Select common elements of academic projects to create a checklist, with options for choosing age range and type of project
	http://pblchecklist.4teachers.org/checklist.shtml
Analog timers showing time remaining	Time Timers available in a variety of sizes and modalities, including wristwatch-type styles. iPad and phone apps and computer options, including smart board applications, are also available
	http://www.timetimer.com/store
Audio prompters	Talking Products' Mini-me is a small device that can record and play 10–20 s audio prompts with the push of a button
	http://www.teachwithsound.com/servlet/StoreFront
	http://www.talkingproducts.com/mini-me-voice-recorder.html
Graphic organizers	Tools4Students (app)
	Kidspiration Maps and Inspiration Maps (app)
	EduPlace, EdHelper, Holt (HRW publishing), TeacherVision, Education Oasis, Thinkport, and Scholastic all have Web sites with graphic organizers, typically by grade level and subject
	http://www.eduplace.com/graphicorganizer/ (English and Spanish)
	http://edhelper.com/teachers/graphic_organizers.htm
	http://my.hrw.com/nsmedia/intgos/html/igo.htm
	http://www.teachervision.com/graphic-organizers/printable/6293.html
	http://www.educationoasis.com/curriculum/graphic_organizers.htm
	http://www.thinkport.org/technology/template.tp
	http://www.scholastic.com/teachers/lesson-plan/graphic-organizers-reading-comprehension
Visual schedules	Choiceworks (app)
	Pinterest and Google images show the variety of options for visual schedules
	Do2Learn (app)
	http://do2learn.com/picturecards/VisualSchedules/index.htm
	http://www.autismschedules.com/Visual-Schedule-Examples.html
	http://www.pbisworld.com/tier-1/visual-schedules/

(continued)

Table 7.1 (continued)

Resource	Description/app
	Web site
Social Stories™	Instructions and programming for creating social stories and downloadable social stories for computer (Pogo Boards, Picto-Selector, Connect ABILITY, LessonPix, and Boardmaker) and apps (StoryMaker for Social Stories, Stories About Me, Stories2Learn, I Create… Social Stories, My Pictures Talk, First Then Visual Schedule, iPrompts)
	http://www.educateautism.com/social-stories.html
	http://www.pbisworld.com/tier-2/social-stories/
	http://www.friendshipcircle.org/blog/2013/02/11/12-computer-programs-websites-and-apps-for-making-social-stories/
Flashcard apps and programs	Flashcards + (app)
	quizlet.com
	studyblue.com
Autism apps	Autism Speaks maintains a Web site listing established and new apps
	http://www.autismspeaks.org/autism-apps?page=1

Individuals who are deficient in executive functioning skills are described as unable to relay the sequence of a story (Cooney and Rood 2011). When those individuals can use a story map to understand and retell a story, their executive functioning skills are improved.

Graphic organizers can easily be generated on a computer (see Table 7.1). Grabe and Jiang (2007) provide many examples of graphic organizers that are made on a computer using text and text boxes. These include cause-and-effect organizers, problem-and-solution organizers, and comparison organizers. In a study done by Bethune and Wood (2013), Wh-question graphic organizers that were made on the computer were given to students to help with their comprehension skills. The paper was divided into four categories and the students were asked to answer the "who," "what," "where," and "why" of a story (Bethune and Wood 2013).

There are also apps for the iPad that can help a student fill out graphic organizers (see Table 7.1). These apps allow learners to choose from multiple graphic organizer templates. The organizers can also be shared through email to their teachers or other peers. Various software programs can also be downloaded onto an iPad. Students are then able to use the iPad to fill out graphic organizers, create outlines, and complete different mind mapping activities.

Checklists

A variation on visual activity schedules for individuals with higher reading levels is a checklist. To help a student stay on task for classroom assignments, different Web sites that facilitate checklist creation can provide some focus. Checklists can help to get ready for an activity (e.g., a list for everything I need to go to lunch, write a paper, or get ready for the bus). The checklist can also help students to monitor their progress and plan for their time accordingly. Checklist applications are available on phones, iPads, and online (see Table 7.1).

Visualizing Tasks (Visual Checklists)

Another application of technology for supporting planning, organization, and self-monitoring is to use cameras on phones and iPads or tablets to capture videos or images of tasks in preparation (get ready—what materials are needed), in progress (what is next, how much time will it take?), and in their finished stages (this is what "done" looks like). On many tablets, a stylus can be used to check off or circle items as they are gathered or finished (Ward and Jacobsen 2014). This technique functions as a visual checklist without the sequence that a visual schedule provides, so it may be more useful for individuals with higher levels of basic executive and cognitive function.

Managing Time

Using technology to support time management skills can be as simple as using a Time Timer or even a regular analog clock (see Table 7.1). Digital clocks and timers do not provide the type of visual support an analog clock face can provide. Applications are available for analog display clocks and timers that can be used on phones, iPads, tablets, computer, wristbands, and smart boards. Even old-fashioned analog clocks can be used with dry-erase markers, stickers, or magnets to help a student visualize how much time a series of tasks will take (Ward and Jacobsen 2014).

Organizing Materials and Tasks

The executive function of organizing can be supported with technology, using cameras to take and post pictures of what an organized desk, closet, room, or workspace looks like. The photograph can be magnified to show details of organization so the student can make their space look like the photograph. Organizational skills involve reading the environment for clues telling a student what needs to happen next and visualizing the future and what will be required to make that future a reality. The visual equivalent of a checklist, pictures of clothes, gear, supplies, etc., can be dragged onto a photograph of the student, workspace, or backpack to show what needs to be gathered for the next activity or task. Real-time apps can also be used to "zoom in" on a scene with an iPhone or iPad to help an individual analyze the environment for clues that tell where to hang up coats, where to turn work in, where to get supplies, how to know how much time is left, where the library books go, where to find help, where to find leisure activities, etc. (Ward and Jacobsen 2014).

Supporting Social and Communication Skills for Learning Through Technology

Technological supports are not limited to strictly academic and executive skills. Technology has been used extensively in individuals with ASD to support social and communication skills, which are also critical for learning.

Social Stories and Social Scripts

Individuals with ASD have difficulties interpreting social cues and responding with or initiating expected behavior in social situations (APA 2013). These difficulties are also possibly explained by poor executive functioning skills. Individuals with ASD can be unaware of the consequences of their actions or find it difficult to understand how their behavior impacts others (Coyne and Rood 2011). Individuals with autism also struggle with taking on multiple perspectives (Sansosti et al. 2004), which would help them to self-monitor their own behavior. One technique that has been used to mitigate these deficits is the intervention of Social Stories[TM].

Social Stories[TM] can help individuals with ASD to understand complex concepts (Sansosti et al. 2004). Social Stories[TM] tells a step-by-step story (with simple text and pictures) about how to act in certain real-life situations. Social stories increase social comprehension because they help those on the spectrum understand what is expected in difficult social situations (Gray 1995). Chan and O'Reilly (2008) showed that social skills are important gateway skills for learning, using social stories as a successful intervention to promote hand-raising behavior by two kindergartners with ASD.

To create a social story, educators must first identify the skill that needs development and break it down into its component steps. It is helpful to gather information from parents and teachers to determine exactly where a student struggles with the task. The story should provide the reader with information about when the social situation might occur, where it might happen, who is involved, what the student is expected to do, and what the consequence will be for the behavior (Gray 2000).

Social Stories[TM] are popular interventions that are easy to share on the Internet (see Table 7.1). As the creator of Social Stories[TM], Carol Gray has typically maintained an Internet presence to help others create and use Social Stories^{TM}. Several educational sites provide instructions, templates, and downloadable Social Stories^{TM} for computers and apps for iPads, phones, and tablets (See Table 7.1). These programs allow users to create stories by organizing different images and your own text. PowerPoint or similar presentation software can also be used to create Social Stories^{TM} on a variety of electronic media, allowing for easy edits or updates as needed. One of the distinct advantages of using technology to create Social Stories^{TM} is the ability to insert actual audio and photographs of people and places into the story. All media platforms allow users to import pictures and record audio for the creation of social stories. The advantages of using Social Stories^{TM} on electronic devices include the ease and speed of creation, adaptability, and the ability to store several stories within a small devices, allowing for easily accessible repetition and viewing as needed.

Social Stories^{TM} are not limited to small format electronics. PowerPoint stories on a smart board can be used to present to the entire class or engage a student with autism in interaction with the story to change learning behaviors (Xin and Sutman 2011). The smart board is a classroom-sized presentation interactive tool that allows the learner to touch and manipulate the pages of the story.

Social scripts are another tool for helping individuals with ASD decipher social situations. Social scripts can be used to encourage conversation between peers (Bourgeois et al. 2008) by providing individuals with a dialogue to employ in different situations, such as meeting someone for the first time or inviting someone over. For individuals needing intervention to develop pragmatic language, audio recordings of social scripts can be used initially as a prompt for basic social language, such as requests. Small, affordable technology such as Talking Products' Mini-Me or similar record-and-play devices can provide a learner-initiated audio prompt for not only social scripts, but actions associated with locations (see Table 7.1). Electronic prompts and scripts themselves can be faded as the student acquires and uses them spontaneously.

Conclusion

Individuals with autism spectrum disorder can be at a disadvantage in the classroom in terms of understanding abstract language and concepts, executive functioning, and social expectations that facilitate learning. There is much that a teacher can do in the classroom to help an individual with ASD. Through social stories, visual supports, and graphic organizers, individuals on the spectrum can better meet the academic demands that are placed upon them. These are tools that do not require intensive training and are not time-consuming, but they can greatly improve the educational experience for an individual with ASD. Technology is readily available to make implementation of these interventions easier than ever before, with the added bonus of more frequent access to intervention and increased social validity.

References

American Psychiatric Association. (2013). *Diagnostic and statistical manual of mental disorders* (5th ed.). Washington, DC: Author.

Banda, D. R., Grimmett, E., & Hart, S. L. (2009). Activity schedules: Helping students with autism spectrum disorders in general education classrooms manage transition issues. *TEACHING Exceptional Children, 41*(4), 16–21.

Baumann, J. F., & Kame'enui, E. J. (1991). Vocabulary instructions: Ode to Voltaire. In J. Flood, J. Jensen, D. Lapp, & J. R. Squire (Eds.), *Handbook of research on teaching the English language arts* (pp. 604–632). New York: Macmillan.

Bethune, K. S., & Wood, C. L. (2013). Effects of wh-questions graphic organizers on reading comprehension skills of students with autism spectrum disorders. *Education and Training in Autism and Developmental Disabilities, 48*(2), 236–244.

Bourgeois, B., Ganz, J. B., Kaylor, M., & Hadden, K. (2008). The impact of social scripts and visual cues on verbal communication in three children with autism spectrum disorder. *Focus on Autism and Other Developmental Disabilities, 23*(2), 79–94.

Broun, L. T. (2004). Teaching students with autistic spectrum disorders to read: A visual approach. *TEACHING Exceptional Children, 36*(4), 36–40.

Bryan, L., & Gast, D. (2000). Teaching on-task and on-schedule behaviors to high functioning children with autism via picture activity schedules. *Journal of Autism and Developmental Disorders, 30*(6), 553–567.

Chan, J. M., & O'Reilly, M. F. (2008). A social stories intervention package for students with autism in inclusive classroom settings. *Journal of Applied Behavior Analysis, 41*(3), 405–409.

Coyne, P., & Rood, K. (2011). Executive function and organization. In P. Coyne (Ed.), *Preparing youth with autism spectrum disorder for adulthood* (pp. 185–226). Oregon: Columbia Regional Program. Retrieved from http://crporegon.org/system/files/documents/AUT_Intro%20to%20toolkit.pdf.

Dakin, S., & Frith, U. (2005). Vagaries of visual perception in autism. *Neuron, 48*(3), 497–507. doi:10.1016/j.neuron.2005.10.018.

Davies, C. (2008). Using visual schedules: A guide for parents. *The Reporter, 14*(1), 18–22.

Dawson, P., & Guare, R. (2010). *Executive skills in children and adolescents: A practical guide to assessment and intervention.* New York: The Guilford Press.

Fisher, J. B., & Schumaker, J. B. (1995). Searching for validated inclusive practices: A review of the literature. *Focus on Exceptional Children, 28*(4), 1–20.

Gately, S. E. (2008). Facilitating reading comprehension for students on the autism spectrum. *TEACHING Exceptional Children, 40*(3), 40–45.

Gray, C. A. (1995). Teaching children with autism to read social situations. In K. A. Quill (Ed.), *Teaching children with autism* (pp. 219–241). New York: Delmar.

Gray, C. A. (2000). *Writing social stories with Carol Gray.* Arlington, TX: Future Horizons.

Hill, E. L., & Bird, C. M. (2006). Executive processes in Asperger syndrome: Patterns of performance in multiple case series. *Neuropsychologia, 44*, 2822–2835.

Hodgdon, L. (2011). *Visual strategies for improving communication.* Troy, MI: QuirkRoberts Publishing.

Jiang, X., & Grabe, W. (2007). Graphic organizers in reading instruction: Research findings and issues. *Reading in a Foreign Language, 19*(1), 34–55.

Jitendra, A. K., Edwards, L. L., Slacks, G., & Jacobson, L. A. (2004). What research says about vocabulary instruction for students with learning disabilities. *Exceptional Children, 70*(3), 299–322.

Kim, A., Vaughn, S., Wanzek, J., & Wei, S. (2004). Graphic organizers and their effects on reading comprehension of students with LD: A synthesis of research. *Journal of Learning Disabilities, 37*(2), 105–118.

King, M. L., Takeguchi, K., Barry, S. E., Rehfeldt, R. A., Boyer, V. E., & Mathews, T. L. (2014). Evaluation of the iPad in the acquisition of requesting skills for children with autism spectrum

disorder. *Research in Autism Spectrum Disorders, 8*(9), 1107–1120. doi:10.1016/j.rasd.2014.
05.011.

Kleinhans, N., Ackshoomof, N., & Delis, D. C. (2005). Executive functions in autism and
Asperger's disorder: Flexibility, fluency, and inhibition. *Developmental Neuropsychology, 27*,
379–401.

Kluth, P., & Darmody-Latham, J. (2003). Beyond sight words: Literacy opportunities for students
with autism. *The Reading Teacher, 56*, 532–535.

McKeon, B., Alpern, C. S., & Zager, D. (2013). Promoting academic engagement for college
students with autism spectrum disorder. *Journal of Postsecondary Education and Disability,
26*(4), 353–366.

Mineo, B. A., Ziegler, W., Gill, S., & Salkin, D. (2009). Engagement with electronic screen media
among students with autism spectrum disorders. *Journal of Autism and Developmental
Disorders, 39*(1), 172–187.

National Professional Development Center in Autism Spectrum Disorders. (n.d.). *Evidence base
for visual supports.* Retrieved December 17, 2014, from http://autismpdc.fpg.unc.edu/sites/
autismpdc.fpg.unc.edu/files/VisualSupports_EvidenceBase.pdf.

National Autism Center. (2009). *National standards report.* Randolph, MA: Author.

National Governors Association Center for Best Practices and Council of Chief State School
Officers. (2010). *Common Core State Standards for English language arts and literacy in
history/social studies, science, and technical subjects.* Washington, DC: Author.

Oelwein, P. (1995). *Teaching reading to children with Down syndrome: A guide for parents and
teachers.* Bethesda, MD: Woodbine House.

Roser, M. E., Aslin, R. N., McKenzie, R., Zahra, D., & Fisher, J. (2014, August 25). Enhanced
visual statistical learning in adults with autism. *Neuropsychology.* doi:10.1037/neu0000137.

Sansosti, F. J., Powell-Smith, K. A., & Kincaid, D. (2004). A research synthesis of social story
interventions for children with autism spectrum disorders. *Focus on Autism and Other
Developmental Disabilities, 19*(4), 194–204.

Scattone, D., Tingstrom, D. H., & Wilczynski, S. M. (2006). Increasing appropriate social
interactions of children with autism spectrum disorders using social stories™. *Focus on Autism
and Other Developmental Disabilities, 21*, 211–222. doi:10.1177/10883576060210040201.

Scruggs, T. E., Brigham, F. J., & Mastropieri, M. A. (2013). Common core science standards:
Implications for students with learning disabilities. *Learning Disabilities Research & Practice,
28*(1), 49–57.

Stringfield, S. G., Luscre, D., & Gast, D. L. (2011). Effects of a story map on accelerated reader
postreading test scores in students with high-functioning autism. *Focus on Autism and Other
Developmental Disabilities, 26*(4), 218–229.

Xin, J. F., & Sutman, F. X. (2011). Using the smart board in teaching social stories to students with
autism. *TEACHING Exceptional Children, 43*(4), 18–24.

Ward, S., & Jacobsen, K. (2014). *Executive function skills in children and adolescents: Assessment
and intervention.* Workshop presentation at the annual meeting of the Utah Psychological
Association, Salt Lake City, UT.

Chapter 8
Do as I'm Doing: Video Modeling and Autism

Teresa A. Cardon

History of Video Modeling

Video modeling (VM) has been used as a tool to support skill development in individuals with autism since the late 1990s. While the medium to record and deliver the video model has rapidly advanced over the past 30 years, driven by drastic changes in technology, the defining characteristics behind VM have remained relatively unchanged. Video modeling is defined as the modeling of a target behavior in a recorded format that results in a video representation via an electronic medium (Ayres and Langone 2005; Bellini and Akullian 2007).

One of the seminal studies involving VM and individuals with autism spectrum disorder (ASD) was designed to compare VM to live modeling, and it was designed to teach a variety of skills (Charlop-Christy et al. 2000). Participants included five children with autism ranging in age from 7 to 11 years. Children with differing functioning levels (e.g., different mental ages, language ages, play skills) were purposefully selected to determine whether VM would be effective across severity levels. All of the children reportedly watched television for at least 30–60 min/day. Different target behaviors were chosen for each child depending on his or her need, as determined by assessments he or she received as part of his or her enrollment in an after-school behavior therapy program. Target behaviors included expressive labeling of emotions, independent play, spontaneous greetings, conversational speech, self-help skills, oral comprehension, cooperative play, and social play. Tasks were randomly assigned to the VM or in vivo condition and ranked by trained college students to be of similar levels of difficulty. Adults who were familiar to the participants provided the model in both the video and live conditions. It is important to note that no prompts or tangible rewards were presented to

T.A. Cardon (✉)
Utah Valley University, Orem, UT, USA
e-mail: Teresa.cardon@uvu.edu

© Springer International Publishing Switzerland 2016
T.A. Cardon (ed.), *Technology and the Treatment of Children with Autism Spectrum Disorder*, Autism and Child Psychopathology Series,
DOI 10.1007/978-3-319-20872-5_8

children during the VM condition, whereas in the in vivo condition, prompts to pay attention and social praise for correct responses were provided.

A multiple baseline design across participants was utilized. Results indicated that children acquired skills faster in the VM condition. Children also generalized target behaviors after VM, but did not generalize target behaviors after live modeling (Charlop-Christy et al. 2000). The total time children spent in the VM condition was 170 min, whereas the total time spent in the live modeling condition was 635 min. In other words, the VM condition was more time- and cost-effective than the in vivo condition. The researchers concluded that VM is an effective technique that can support skill development in children with ASD. Since that time, VM has been used to teach a variety of skills to children, adolescents, and adults with autism across multiple contexts.

A meta-analysis analyzing the effectiveness of VM as an intervention tool for children with autism was conducted on 23 studies published between 1987 and 2005 (Bellini an Akullian 2007). A total of 73 participants, ranging in age from 3 to 20 years, were included. The average number of VM sessions conducted was 9.5 with the average duration of each clip being reported as 3 min. Percentage of non-overlapping data points (PND) were analyzed across the three dependent variable categories and revealed that the highest intervention effects were found for functional skills, followed by social communication skills and then behavioral skills (Bellini and Akullian 2007). The researchers concluded that VM is an effective intervention strategy to teach skills to children with ASD, and skills are both maintained and generalized after treatment is concluded (Bellini and Akullian 2007).

Video modeling has been demonstrated to be an effective technique in schools and the community. Research has indicated that educators can apply VM in school settings. Bellini and Akullian (2007) reported that the majority of the studies they reviewed took place in school settings. In school settings, VM has been used to increase academic skills (e.g., Delano 2007; Kinney et al. 2003; Hitchcock et al. 2003), decrease disruptive behaviors (Apple et al. 2005; Buggey 2005), and increase social interactions (e.g., Cihak et al. 2009; Nikopoulos and Keenan 2003; Wert and Neisworth 2003). In general, the focus on community applications of VM has included increasing appropriate behaviors and effective transitions (e.g., Schreibman et al. 2000), but community applications have also focused on daily living skills by helping individuals with ASD choose items to purchase at a store (Alacantara 1994; Haring et al. 1995) and independently purchase items (Mechling et al. 2005).

Video modeling is an effective strategy to promote skill acquisition in children with ASD because they (a) are partial to visual stimuli (e.g., Kinney et al. 2003), (b) can focus more efficiently on restricted fields due to issues with overselectivity (i.e., attending to non-relevant stimuli; e.g., Corbett 2003), (c) often have exceptional memories and are skilled echoers (e.g., Charlop and Milstein 1989), and (d) appear to avoid face-to-face interactions (e.g., Charlop-Christy et al. 2000). In addition, VM has several practical advantages for use as an intervention tool, such as (a) the capacity to present an assortment of examples, (b) concise control over the modeling process, (c) exact repetition and reuse of video clips, and (d) cost and time efficiency of intervention (Corbett 2003).

Theoretical Support for Video Modeling

As mentioned previously, VM has been used to teach a variety of skills to children with autism including imitation, play skills, self-help skills, and social skills (e.g., Ayres and Langone 2005; Cardon 2012; Cardon and Wilcox 2011; D'Ateno et al. 2003). It has been suggested that VM supports the development of observational learning, specifically the cognitive and behavioral changes humans experience as a result of watching or observing others involved in similar actions (Bandura 1977; Corbett 2003). According to Bandura, observational learning, or social learning theory, is critical to the development and survival of human beings as we learn what we should and should not do by observing events that occur around us. For observational learning to be successful, four components must be present: attention, retention, production, and motivation. We pay attention to activities that are modeled and then retain that information to utilize later. The actions that are observed can then be imitated (Bandura 1977). Although every action that is observed does not translate into perfect imitation, the awareness of the action has been created. Further, Bandura posited that the accuracy of imitative acts is reliant on positive reinforcement and continued input from others. The motivational factors that shape imitation in observational learning differentiate Bandura's theory from Piaget's in that Piaget attributes the desire to imitate to intrinsic needs as opposed to external factors.

A relatively new theory, proposed by researchers working at the Medical Investigation of Neurodevelopmental Disorders (MIND) Institute at UC Davis, implicates the visual attention differences present in children with autism (Vivanti et al. 2008). Researchers wanted to determine what children with autism look at when an imitative act is demonstrated. They believed that patterns in children's visual attention could provide insight into how actions are encoded and ultimately which acts are imitated based on those patterns (Vivanti et al. 2008). The study included 18 children with autism and 13 children with typical development. It is important to note that all of the imitative acts presented to the participants were through prerecorded video clips. No live models were used. When controlling for the language level of the participants, researchers discovered that both groups more accurately imitated actions involving objects than those involving gestures. In addition, both groups visually attended to the action region (region where the action was performed) more during tasks that involved object imitation; however, differences were found between the two groups with regard to visual attention to the face region (area of the face of the demonstrator performing the action). Specifically, the children with autism looked at the face region less than half the time the typical children spent looking at the face region. The researchers proposed that the decreased attention to the face region could provide specific insight into the relationship between imitation deficits and social deficits present in children with autism. Future research into the visual attention skills of children with autism and the impact that visual attention has on imitation is necessary to determine the accuracy of the visual attention theory.

In summary, VM is thought to work as an intervention for children with autism because of several specific elements. When used as an intervention tool, VM capitalizes on the visual preferences (e.g., television watching, lining up toys to view them, repeatedly watching objects spin) exhibited in many children with autism (Corbett 2003; Kinney et al. 2003). Further, the screen offers a restricted field of vision and can therefore focus a child's attention on relevant stimuli while decreasing their tendency to attend to irrelevant stimuli (e.g., Charlop-Christy et al. 2000; Corbett 2003). Screens are highly motivating, and reinforcement to attend to the task is built right in (Corbett 2003). And finally, children with autism attend for longer periods of time to screens as opposed to live presentations of information (Cardon and Azuma 2012; Vivanti et al. 2008).

Parameters of Video Modeling and Autism

As is evidenced by the numerous studies, VM is an effective intervention tool that can be used to teach play skills, language skills, self-help skills, social communication skills, functional daily living skills, academic skills, and appropriate behaviors. In addition, a number of reviews and meta-analyses have been conducted that identify the ability of children with ASD to maintain learned skills and to generalize those skills to new, previously undeveloped behaviors (Bellini and Akullian 2007; Ayres and Langone 2005; McCoy and Hermansen 2007; Gelbar et al. 2012). With regard to additional parameters of VM, however, there are several other components that should be considered.

Original research surrounding VM and autism looked at school-age and adolescent children to determine whether it was an effective intervention tool, particularly when targeting self-help skills or social skills (e.g., Charlop and Milstein 1989; Charlop-Christy et al. 2000; Nikopoulos and Keenan 2003). While seminal studies reported that older children with ASD responded positively to VM, more recent research has targeted younger children with ASD. In 2011, Cardon and Wilcox demonstrated that VM to teach object imitation was effective for children with ASD as young as 20 months of age. Further, very young children with ASD responded to VM used to teach object imitation, self-help skills, gestural imitation, and verbal imitation (Cardon 2012, 2013). Given the wide age ranges of children who respond to VM and the rapid response times that have been reported, introducing it as an early technique to support skill development is recommended.

In the home environment, emerging research has demonstrated that VM can be used by caregivers to teach a number of skills. Specifically, caregivers have been able to effectively create their own video models at home in order to teach fine motor skills (e.g., cutting with scissors and correct pencil grip), self-help skills (e.g., bed making), play skills (e.g., pretend play with a doll, puzzle completion), and social skills such as responding with, "No thank you" when offered an unpreferred food item (Cardon 2012). Similarly, VM has been utilized to teach children with autism how to interact with their siblings. Research conducted by Reagon et al. (2006) determined that children with ASD could be taught via VM to interact with their siblings during several different pretend play scenarios (e.g., cowboy dress-ups, playing teacher). It is recommended that VM be considered as a possible intervention technique across settings with a variety of individuals.

As described, VM can support skill development in both younger and older children across settings; however, there are some advanced parameters of the video model that should be considered. To begin with, some children have been able to successfully learn fine motor skills, such as cutting and tracing (Cardon 2012) using VM; however, recent research has indicated that the size of the screen may impact skill acquisition when attempting to learn fine motor tasks. Specifically, researchers analyzed screen size to determine whether the size of the screen used to present the video model impacted skill acquisition (Mechling and Ayres 2012; Mechling and Youhouse 2012). Results indicated that fine motor tasks increased regardless of screen size; however, more correct responses resulted from the use of a larger screen, particularly if an intellectual disability was present. It is important to note, however, that to date there is no research to indicate any significant differences between smartphones, tablets, or iPod touches with regard to skill acquisition and VM.

Another element of the video model that is helpful to consider is the use of a verbal description or a verbal narrative as an accompanying element of the video model. While this seems like an obvious parameter when teaching social communication skills via VM, it is also beneficial when teaching other target skills. For example, children learning pretend play skills, gestures, and self-help skills via VM have demonstrated increased verbal language skills after exposure to the video model (e.g., Boudreau and D'Entremont 2010; Cardon and Wilcox 2011; Cardon 2012; McDonald et al. 2005). Given that verbal language may be a pivotal component of VM intervention, it is recommended that verbal descriptions or narratives be included along with the video model.

It has been recognized that children with ASD respond well when increased levels of motivation are present (Koegel and Koegel 2006). It has also been suggested that the nature of VM increases motivation because of the presence of the electronic medium (i.e., tablet, smartphone; Corbett 2003) and that children may respond to VM because highly preferred items are being utilized during the intervention (Carr et al. 2000; Mechling et al. 2006). A recent study analyzed skill acquisition during VM when both preferred and non-preferred items were present (Robinson and Cardon 2012). Results indicated that participants imitated actions with both preferred and non-preferred objects and, contrary to the previous research, participants imitated actions with non-preferred items more consistently than preferred items. In other words, imitation occurred at high rates regardless of item preference. It may be beneficial to include novel actions and objects when implementing VM.

Often when describing the how-to aspects of VM, researchers take care to describe how to create videos that are free of visual and auditory distractions, but research on the specific requirements of the video model is limited. A recent study looked at one element of possible visual distractions that may be present in a video model (Gilbert and Cardon 2012). The researchers recorded models performing a target action with an object in front of a green screen. Three separate visual backgrounds were then embedded over the green screen: a plain background, a distracting background, and a moving background. In other words, the visual foreground of the video remained the same, while the background visually changed. Children with autism were shown the video clips in random order. All of the children that participated were able to imitate the target action with the object regardless of what background was present in the video. While further research is needed, the willingness that children with ASD have to imitate what they see on a video, be it preferred or non-preferred, and distracting or not, is an important component to take into consideration.

Video Modeling Implementation

In general, children with ASD that have shown a prior preference for visual stimuli or visual learning may respond better to VM as an intervention technique (Sherer et al. 2001). There are typically three types of VM that have been used to teach a variety of skills: classic video modeling, point of view, and video self-modeling.

Classic VM involves filming a model performing a target action. The video captures the model and the target action being completed correctly. The video is then presented to the child with autism. The child watches the video and is then given a chance to perform the task. As mentioned previously, classic VM has been used effectively to teach play skills, social skills, self-help skills, daily living skills, language skills, and academic skills.

Point of view video modeling (POVM) involves filming from the point of view of the model, often only showing their hands close-up as they complete a task. This type of VM has been effectively used to teach toy play to preschoolers (Hine and Wolery 2006), self-help skills, such as dressing (Norman et al. 2001), and daily living skills (Shipley-Benamou et al. 2002; Sigafoos et al. 2005). To some degree, POVM was helpful in supporting social behaviors in preschool and school-age children with ASD (Tetreault and Lerman 2010).

Video self-modeling (VSM) involves recording the child with autism performing the target skill multiple times and then editing the recordings to create a final product in which the child is shown to be demonstrating the skill correctly. The child only views the video of himself or herself performing the task correctly. VSM is more time-consuming and requires more technical skills because of the editing requirements; however, it has been found to be effective when teaching a variety of skills. Specifically, VSM can improve language and social skills, (e.g., Bellini and Akullian 2007; Lantz 2005), on-task behavior (Coyle and Cole 2004), and adherence to classroom expectations (e.g., Lang et al. 2009; Cihak 2011). A number of reviews and meta-analyses have been conducted to determine whether the type of VM used (i.e., classic vs. self versus point of view) impacts effectiveness. To date, no differences have been found and all types of VM have met criteria for evidence-based practice (Horner et al. 2005).

With regard to the age of the individual acting as the video model, research indicates that siblings, peers, and adults all make effective models (e.g., Bellini and Akullian 2007; Cardon 2012). That being said, working with more mature models may take less time and training, making it more cost-effective. While the majority of VM research focuses on a one-on-one session when showing the child with ASD the video model, there is emerging research that indicates that VM can be used effectively in group settings (Kroeger et al. 2007; Plavnick et al. 2013). The flexibility within VM as an intervention contributes to its usability and practicality.

While steps to creating a video model used to require a certain level of technical ability, with the introduction of smartphones and tablet computers, the technical skills to create a video model are almost universal. While these steps must be adapted to the type of device being used and the type of video model being created (i.e., classic vs. self vs. point of view), the basics steps are as follows:

1. Determine the target behavior you would like to focus on. The target behavior should be developmentally appropriate given the child's age and stage.
2. Determine who you would like to film as the video model.
3. Determine how you would like to film the video (i.e., classic vs. self vs. point of view).
4. Have the model practice the target behavior several times. Creating a task analysis, or a list of the necessary steps, can be helpful. It is helpful to have the model verbalize, or describe, what they are doing. Or, think about what a child would say naturally when completing the task. Verbalizing during the video model is important because children often start to imitate what they hear and see!
5. Practice filming the model performing the target behavior with the video application on your smartphone or tablet.
6. Watch the video to make sure that you have captured every step of the target behavior and to make sure that the sound and picture quality is clear.
7. Present the video model to the child in an environment that is appropriate and conducive to their learning. Be sure to have any objects or materials that the child will need to complete the task nearby.
8. Play the video model for the child one time. If an object is required for the target behavior, have it sitting nearby where they can reach it or be sure to immediately hand them the item when the video is over.
9. If the child imitates, praise them! If the child does not imitate, play the video for them again.
10. If the child has three unsuccessful attempts, feel free to physically prompt the child to perform the target behavior. A physical prompt can help them understand what is required of them and may increase their level of success.

Children with ASD often like to watch the videos over and over again. As long as they are also performing the target behavior, watching the videos only reinforces the skill. They can watch the videos several times a day or several times a week. As mentioned previously, researchers have discovered that children can learn multiple skills via VM at the same time, so feel free to choose several target behaviors at once. Not all children respond to VM, but those that do tend to respond quickly (Charlop-Christy et al. 2000; Cardon 2012). If a child is struggling, you can always back off to one skill or review the video to see whether something needs to be rerecorded.

Video modeling is a well-researched intervention and can be used by caregivers and clinicians alike. It is a highly effective and efficient tool that supports a range of target behaviors in an assortment of environments. Over the past 30 years, VM has become more commonplace and it is a powerful tool that continues to enrich the lives of children with autism.

References

Alcantara, P. R. (1994). Effects of videotape instructional package on purchasing skills of children with autism. *Exceptional Children, 61*(1), 40–55.

Apple, A. L., Billingsley, F., Schwartz, I. S., & Carr, E. G. (2005). Effects of video modeling alone and with self-management on compliment-giving behaviors of children with high-functioning ASD. *Journal of Positive Behavior Interventions, 7*(1), 33–46.

Ayres, K. M., & Langone, J. (2005). Intervention and instruction with video for students with autism: A review of the literature. *Education and Training in Developmental Disabilities, 40*(2), 183–196.

Bandura, A. (1977). Self-efficacy: Toward a unifying theory of behavioral change. *Psychological Review, 84*, 191–215.

Bellini, S., & Akullian, J. (2007). A meta-analysis of video modeling and video self-modeling interventions for children and adolescents with autism spectrum disorders. *Exceptional Children, 73*(3), 264–287.

Boudreau, E., & D'Entremont, B. (2010). Improving the pretend play skills of preschoolers with autism spectrum disorders: The effects of video modeling. *Journal of Developmental and Physical Disabilities, 22*(4), 415–431.

Buggey, T. (2005). Video self-modeling applications with students with autism spectrum disorder in a small private school setting. *Focus on Autism and Other Developmental Disabilities, 20*(1), 52–63.

Cardon, T. (2013). Video modeling imitation training to support gestural imitation acquisition in young children with ASD. *Speech, Language and Hearing, 16*(4), 227–238.

Cardon, T. (2012). Teaching caregivers to implement video modeling imitation training via iPad for their children with autism. *Research in Autism Spectrum Disorders, 6*, 1389–1400.

Cardon, T., & Azuma, T. (2012). Visual attending preferences in children with autism spectrum disorders: A comparison between live and video presentation modes. *Research in Autism Spectrum Disorders, 6*, 1061–1067.

Cardon, T. A., & Wilcox, M. J. (2011). Promoting imitation in young children with autism: A comparison of reciprocal imitation training and video modeling. *Journal of Autism and Developmental Disorders, 41*(5), 654–677.

Carr, J. E., Nicolson, A. C., & Higbee, T. S. (2000). Evaluation of a brief multiple-stimulus preference assessment in a naturalistic context. *Journal of Applied Behavior Analysis, 33*(3), 353–357.

Cihak, D. F. (2011). Comparing pictorial and video modeling activity schedules during transitions for students with autism spectrum disorders. *Research in Autism Spectrum Disorders, 5*(1), 433–441.

Cihak, D., Fahrenkrog, C., Ayres, K. M., & Smith, C. (2009). The use of video modeling via a video iPod and a system of least prompts to improve transitional behaviors for students with autism spectrum disorders in the general education classroom. *Journal of Positive Behavior Interventions, 12*(2), 103–115.

Charlop-Christy, M. H., Le, L., & Freeman, K. (2000). A comparison of video modeling with in vivo modeling for teaching children with autism. *Journal of Autism and Developmental Disorders, 30*, 537–552.

Charlop, M. H., & Milstein, J. P. (1989). Teaching autistic children conversational speech using video modeling. *Journal of Applied Behavior Analysis, 22*(3), 275–285.

Corbett, B. A. (2003). Video modeling: A window into the world of autism. *The Behavior Analyst Today, 4*, 88–96.

Coyle, C., & Cole, P. (2004). A videotaped self-modeling and self-monitoring treatment program to decrease off-task behaviour in children with autism. *Journal of Intellectual and Developmental Disability, 29*(1), 3–15.

D'Ateno, P., Mangiapanello, K., & Taylor, B. A. (2003). Using video modeling to teach complex play sequences to a preschooler with autism. *Journal of Positive Behavior Interventions, 5*, 5–11.

Delano, M. E. (2007). Improving written language performance of adolescents with Asperger syndrome. *Journal of Applied Behavior Analysis, 40*(2), 345–351.

Gelbar, N. W., Anderson, C., McCarthy, S., & Buggey, T. (2012). Video self-modeling as an intervention strategy for individuals with autism spectrum disorders. *Psychology in the Schools, 49*(1), 15–22.

Gilbert, A., & Cardon, T. (December, 2012). Parameters of Video Modeling and its Impact on Imitation Skills in a Child with Autism Spectrum Disorder. Inland Northwest Research Symposium, Spokane, WA.

Haring, T., Breen, C., Weiner, J., Kennedy, C., & Bednersh, E. (1995). Using videotape modeling to facilitate generalized purchasing skills. *Journal of Behavioral Education, 5*, 29–53.

Hine, J. F., & Wolery, M. (2006). Using point-of-view video modeling to teach play to preschoolers with autism. *Topics in Early Childhood Special Education, 26*(2), 83–93.

Hitchcock, C. H., Dowrick, P. W., & Prater, M. A. (2003). Video self-modeling intervention in school-based settings a review. *Remedial and Special Education, 24*(1), 36–45.

Horner, R. H., Carr, E. G., Halle, J., McGee, G., Odom, S., & Wolery, M. (2005). The use of single subject research to identify evidence-based practice in special education. *Exceptional Children, 71*, 165–179.

Kinney, E. M., Vedora, J., & Stromer, R. (2003). Computer-presented video models to teach generative spelling to a child with an autism spectrum disorder. *Journal of Positive Behavior Interventions, 5*(1), 22–29.

Koegel, R., & Koegel, L. (2006). *Pivotal response treatments for autism* (pp. 141–159). Baltimore, MD: Paul H. Brookes Publishing Co.

Kroeger, K. A., Schultz, J. R., & Newsom, C. (2007). A comparison of two group-delivered social skills programs for young children with autism. *Journal of Autism and Developmental Disorders, 37*(5), 808–817.

Lang, R., Shogren, K. A., Machalicek, W., Rispoli, M., O'Reilly, M., Baker, S., & Regester, A. (2009). Video self-modeling to teach classroom rules to two students with Asperger's. *Research in Autism Spectrum Disorders, 3*, 483–488.

Lantz, J. F. (2005). Using video self-modeling to increase the prosocial behavior of children with autism and their siblings. Unpublished doctoral dissertation, Indiana University, Bloomington.

McCoy, K., & Hermansen, E. (2007). Video modeling for individuals with autism: A review of model types and effects. *Education and Treatment of Children, 30*(4), 183–213.

MacDonald, R., Clark, M., Garrigan, E., & Vangala, M. (2005). Using video modeling to teach pretend play to children with autism. *Behavioral Interventions, 20*(4), 225–238.

Mechling, L. C., & Ayres, K. M. (2012). A comparative study: Completion of fine motor office related tasks by high school students with autism using video models on large and small screen sizes. *Journal of Autism and Developmental Disorders, 42*, 2364–2373.

Mechling, L. C., Gast, D., & Cronin, B. (2006). The effects of presenting high-preference items, paired with choice, via computer-based video programming on task completion of students with autism. *Focus on Autism and Other Developmental Disabilities, 21*(7), 7–13.

Mechling, L. C., Pridgen, L. S., & Cronin, B. A. (2005). Computer-based video instruction to teach students with intellectual disabilities to verbally respond to questions and make purchases in fast food restaurants. *Education and Training in Developmental Disabilities, 40*(1), 47–59.

Mechling, L. C., & Youhouse, I. R. (2012). Comparison of task performance by students with autism and moderate intellectual disabilities when presenting video models on large and small screen sizes. *Journal of Special Education Technology, 27*(1), 1–14.

Nikopoulos, C. K., & Keenan, M. (2003). Promoting social initiation in children with autism using video modeling. *Behavioral Interventions, 18*(2), 87–108.

Norman, J. M., Collins, B. C., & Schuster, J. W. (2001). Using an instructional package including video technology to teach self-help skills to elementary students with mental disabilities. *Journal of Special Education Technology, 16*(3), 5–18.

Plavnick, J. B., Sam, A. M., Hume, K., & Odom, S. L. (2013). Effects of video-based group instruction for adolescents with autism spectrum disorder. *Exceptional Children, 80*(1), 67–83.

Reagon, K. A., Higbee, T. S., & Endicott, K. (2006). Teaching pretend play skills to a student with autism using video modeling with a sibling as model and play partner. *Education and Treatment of Children, 25*, 517.

Robinson, K., & Cardon, T. (December, 2012). Assessment of Video Modeling Imitation Skills Using Preferred and Non-preferred Toys in a Child with Autism Spectrum Disorder. Inland Northwest Research Symposium, Spokane, WA.

Schreibman, L., Whalen, C., & Stahmer, A. C. (2000). The use of video priming to reduce disruptive transition behavior in children with autism. *Journal of Positive Behavior Interventions, 2*(1), 3–11.

Sherer, M., Pierce, K. L., Paredes, S., Kisacky, K. L., Ingersoll, B., & Schreibman, L. (2001). Enhancing conversational skills in children with autism via video technology: Which is better? "Self" or "other" as model? *Behavior Modification, 25*, 140–158.

Shipley-Benamou, R., Lutzker, J. R., & Taubman, M. (2002). Teaching daily living skills to children with autism through instructional video modeling. *Journal of Positive Behavior Interventions, 4*(3), 166–177.

Sigafoos, J., O'Reilly, M., Cannella, H., Upadhyaya, M., Edrisinha, C., Lancioni, G. E., & Young, D. (2005). Computer-presented video prompting for teaching microwave oven use to three adults with developmental disabilities. *Journal of Behavioral Education, 14*(3), 189–201.

Tetreault, A. S., & Lerman, D. C. (2010). Teaching social skills to children with autism using point-of-view video modeling. *Education and Treatment of Children, 33*(3), 395–419.

Vivanti, G., Nadig, A., Ozonoff, S., & Rogers, S. J. (2008). What do children with autism attend to during imitation tasks? *Journal of Experimental Child Psychology, 101*(3), 186–205.

Wert, B. Y., & Neisworth, J. T. (2003). Effects of video self-modeling on spontaneous requesting in children with autism. *Journal of Positive Behavior Interventions, 5*(1), 30–34.

Chapter 9
Tapping into Technical Talent: Using Technology to Facilitate Personal, Social, and Vocational Skills in Youth with Autism Spectrum Disorder (ASD)

Marissa Lynn Diener, Cheryl A. Wright, Scott D. Wright and Laura Linnell Anderson

Participation in extracurricular activities is related to better outcomes for neuro-typical youth in a number of domains, including school functioning and psycho-social development. However, parents of youth with autism spectrum disorder (ASD) report that their children often have difficulty in traditional extracurricular activities and may not enjoy or experience the same levels of success as their neurotypical peers in these activities. To address this need, we have developed a technology-based summer and after-school program that teaches youth with ASD software skills that enable them to create 3D designs. The program involves peers with ASD who have interests in technology, family members, and supportive mentoring adults. Our preliminary results indicate that by focusing on the talents, strengths, and interests of youth with ASD, rather than on remediating deficits, we made a difference in 3 domains: increased self-esteem and confidence for youth, enhanced social engagement with peers and family members, and vocational exploration and aspirations.

This chapter describes an innovative out-of-school program designed to address gaps in vocational preparation for adolescents and young adults on the autism spectrum. The program represents a shift from a deficit-based, biomedical approach to autism; instead, it is built on a positive youth development framework to create a technology program that builds on the strengths and interests of youth with autism to promote vocational exploration, software skill development, and social engagement (Dawes and Larson 2011; Hansen and Larson 2007; Ramey and Rose-Krasnor 2012). The program is grounded in a community-based participatory research model (see Wright et al. 2014) and is backed by social entrepreneurs and corporate leaders in the technology industry.

Approximately 50,000 young adults with ASD turn 18 years each year (Donovan and Zucker 2010). These young adults may face social isolation,

M.L. Diener (✉) · C.A. Wright · S.D. Wright · L.L. Anderson
University of Utah, Salt Lake City, UT, USA
e-mail: marissa.diener@fcs.utah.edu

© Springer International Publishing Switzerland 2016
T.A. Cardon (ed.), *Technology and the Treatment of Children with Autism Spectrum Disorder*, Autism and Child Psychopathology Series,
DOI 10.1007/978-3-319-20872-5_9

underemployment and unemployment, and limited post-secondary opportunities as they age out of the education system (Wei et al. 2014). Calls to action to address the needs of these youth indicate that there are few interventions or programs to support vocational preparation in this population (Levy and Perry 2011; McDonald and Machalicek 2013). The current focus in autism is an emphasis on early intervention, in order to remediate the deficits associated with the disorder, and in fact, these early interventions show positive effects on children's development (Dawson and Bernier 2013; Reichow 2012). In comparison, few interventions focus on vocational interventions for adolescents or young adults with ASD (Taylor et al. 2012). Yet greater vocational independence and engagement is related to subsequent reductions in autism symptoms and maladaptive behaviors and improvements in activities in daily living for adults with ASD (Taylor and Seltzer 2011).

The positive youth developmental approach arose out of an increasing recognition that in order to understand and support life span development, rather than focus more exclusively on developmental psychopathology, research must focus on the strengths and skills of youth and include the person-in-context (Benson et al. 2006; Larson 2000; Ramey and Rose-Krasnor 2012). The positive youth development approach argues that adolescents need opportunities to be motivated, to want to participate in an activity, and to be invested it, rather than to be motivated by rewards or anticipated rewards (Larson 2000). Thus, rather than pulling youth toward particular paths of development, they need to be intrinsically motivated to engage over time in activities toward a goal (Larson 2000). Larson (2000) defines initiative as the willingness to devote sustained effort over time even in the face of challenge to achieve a goal. Voluntary structured activities, such as extracurricular school activities, hobbies, sports, and school activities, often provide opportunities for initiative, because they are often intrinsically motivating and engaging, and participants often regulate their own behavior in pursuit of a goal. These processes promote skills and competence, while also promoting self-regulatory processes (Larson 2000).

Conceptualizations of ideal youth development programs provide three characteristics: (1) opportunities for participation and leadership in family, school, and community; (2) an emphasis on life skills; and (3) supportive adult–youth relationships (Lerner 2004). Structured youth activities give youth opportunities to exert control, learn skills, and be intrinsically motivated (Larson 2000). These activities are related to positive development because they provide opportunities to develop skills, interests, a sense of purpose, and supportive adult relationships (Ramey and Rose-Krasnor 2012). Not only are youth impacted by these structured activities, they impact the communities and organizations within which they act, making the influences bidirectional. Moments of engagement provide meaning, resulting in greater involvement and investment in an interest area (Hidi and Renninger 2006). Interest influences attention, goals, and levels of learning (see Hidi and Renninger 2006).

Despite the importance of these activities for skill building and positive development, children with ASD show restricted participation in structured extracurricular activities in comparison with peers with other disabilities such as health impairments or hearing impairments (Wagner et al. 2002). For example, research indicates that children with high functioning ASD participated in a narrower range of activities, less frequently, and with a narrower group of peers (Hochhauser and Engel-Yeger 2010). They were more likely to experience leisure activities at home than were typically developing peers (Hochhauser and Engel-Yeger 2010). Only 18 % had participated in a school-sponsored group in the previous year, although more (42 %) had participated in a community-sponsored group activity in the previous year. The lower participation rates are likely due to complex factors, including both student and situational factors.

The Role of Technology and Positive Development for Youth with ASD

One potential for engaging youth with autism involves technology and electronic screen media (ESM). Parents often report that children with autism are drawn to and have a propensity for computer technology and other forms of ESM (Buggey 2005; Charlop-Christy and Daneshvar 2003; Heiman et al. 1995; Nally et al. 2000). In fact, it has been argued that ESM helps those with ASDs focus their attention because the constrained viewing area limits the attentional frame (Charlop-Christy and Daneshvar 2003). Furthermore, Bosseler and Massaro (2003) suggested that computer characteristics such as controllability and adaptability can be reassuring for youth with ASD. Because ESM, including computer software, puts the user in charge, rather than making demands on the individual, and does not necessarily involve interference from other people, it is often appealing to individuals with autism (Bernard-Opitz et al. 2001; Shipley-Benamou et al. 2002). In fact, youth with ASDs often appear to be more attentive to computer programs than to individuals (Moore and Calvert 2000). Moore and Calvert (2000) demonstrated that children with ASD learned more from a computer condition than they did in a teacher-only condition. Furthermore, parents and caregivers of children with ASD indicated that their children spent more leisure time engaged with ESM than any other activity (Shane and Albert 2008). Thus, programs that capitalize on the interests of youth with autism by including technology may be beneficial.

In fact, the use of interactive technologies for individuals with ASD has grown dramatically over the last decade (Kientz et al. 2014; Knight et al. 2013; Porayska-Pomsta et al. 2012; Wainer and Ingersoll 2011) and has become increasingly important, as reflected in the chapters in this book. ESM approaches have proliferated, taking many forms, including video modeling and virtual reality (Cardon 2013; Cardon and Wilcox 2011; Grynszpan et al. 2008; Pennington 2010; Ploog et al. 2013). Video modeling, which provides videotaped examples of models (self, peers, adults, and Disney characters) demonstrating various behaviors, has been used widely. These approaches offer many advantages, including maintenance of fidelity, reduced need for language-based approaches, consistency in delivery, and the ability to present dangerous or impractical scenarios with no real-world consequences (Mineo et al. 2009; Parsons and Cobb 2005). The focus of the research with technology has typically been to develop and evaluate technologically supported interventions or diagnostic aids (e.g., Golan et al. 2010).

In addition to being drawn to ESM, including software programs, visual–spatial skills are often, though not always, a strength of people with autism (Grandin 1995; Kennedy and Banks 2011). One study demonstrated that children with ASD showed more unique designs than typically developing children, using 3D shapes, suggesting strengths in their visual–spatial creativity (Grandin 2009; Roskos-Ewoldsen et al. 2008; see also Kaldy et al. 2013; Schmidt et al. 2012). The literature documents frequent accounts of artists with autism (Mottron and Belleville 1993; Selfe 1983). One study demonstrated that individuals with ASD showed superior performance in map learning (Caron et al. 2004). Individuals with ASD also often appear to be above average on systemizing, or analyzing and constructing rule-based systems (Baron-Cohen 2006; Baron-Cohen et al. 2009; Caldwell-Harris and Jordan 2014; Gonzalez et al. 2013). Given these systemizing strengths, it is not surprising that individuals with autism may gravitate toward STEM occupations (Baron-Cohen et al. 2007). Individuals with autism appear to have an affinity for science, math, engineering, and technology (STEM) careers (Spek and Velderman 2013). Despite low college enrollment rates overall, individuals with ASD are more likely to persist in college and also more likely to transfer from a 2-year community college to a 4-year university if they are a STEM major than a non-STEM major (Wei et al. 2014). Compared to other students with disabilities as well as students in the general population, young adults with ASD are more likely to major in STEM fields, especially science or computer science (Chen and Weko 2009; Wei et al. 2013).

The program described here represents a shift in the typical approach, adopting conceptual models from the positive youth development movement of how to create meaningful, engaged learning. The program described here uses engaging mentors that model risk taking, humor, and enthusiasm (Shernoff 2012). The importance of an activity that is meaningful and intrinsically motivating has been noted. Effective interventions focus on special interests, leverage visual–spatial abilities in youth, and complement school curricula (Khowaja and Salim 2013). One specific interest of many youth with autism is technology. The central component of the program discussed here involves free 3D design software called SketchUp Make. Anecdotal evidence suggests that some individuals with ASDs have a propensity for this computer program (Kalb 2009), and our research supports this conclusion (Wright et al. 2011).

NeuroVersity Program

What Is NeuroVersity?

The technology program described here, called NeuroVersity, is designed primarily for students with high functioning autism (HFA) in an effort to provide these students with opportunities to develop and demonstrate technology skills, socialize

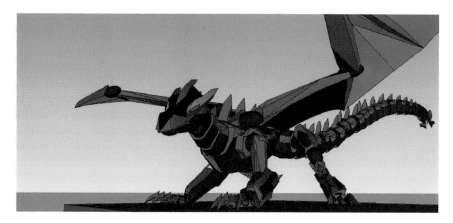

Fig. 9.1 Dragon created in SketchUp by student in Salt Lake City, summer 2014

with peers, and explore vocational interests. During the one-week workshops, students learn how to use SketchUp Make to create 3D designs based on their individual interests. SketchUp Make is a free visual–spatial design program used by civil and mechanical engineers, architects, film and video game designers, interior designers, and other professionals who use computer-based modeling. The software is used to create 3D models of physical spaces, buildings, and objects that can be rotated, animated, and viewed from multiple angles (see Figs. 9.1 and 9.2).

Students in the NeuroVersity program are able to design whatever interests them, and also have access to the 3D Warehouse, an online repository of free models that can be downloaded and shared. Summer workshops occur over 1–2 weeks for 3 h per day, Monday through Friday. The summer workshops are followed up in the fall by an after-school program, which follows a similar format. The workshops are led by a professional who works in a field that uses SketchUp

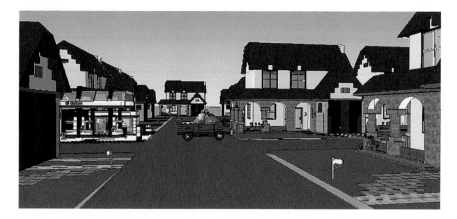

Fig. 9.2 Lego Town created by a student in The Dalles, OR, summer 2013

and acts as a mentor to the students in creative design. The mentor reinforces the real-world application of the design program daily.

NeuroVersity's primary goal is to provide students with opportunities to use their strengths in an educational setting to learn and enhance a variety of skills. The program follows a structured schedule beginning with an ice-breaker activity such as legos while waiting for all students to arrive. Next, the mentor provides about 20 min of instruction in the SketchUp tools used to create the designs. Students are then given about an hour to experiment with and master those tools as they create their own 3D design based on their own interests. The SketchUp mentor provides individual feedback and support during group work time, and two facilitators, professionals or paraprofessionals who work with youth with ASD, provide positive behavior support throughout the session. After a short break, students project their designs on a large screen in order to share and discuss them with the group if they choose. Family members are encouraged to attend these presentations at the end of each session in order to provide positive feedback and see what the students have accomplished. At the end of the week-long workshop, students share their projects with their group, their families, significant others, and community members. This final presentation and celebration provides an opportunity for the students to show off their skills. The summer workshops are followed by a weekly after-school program, which follows a similar format of SketchUp lesson, design time, and presentations. The NeuroVersity team also coordinates family events and community workshops in which students teach community members SketchUp and facilitates student presentations to peers in their classrooms.

What Makes NeuroVersity Different?

NeuroVersity is unique in several ways: It provides a student-centered, interest-based approach (Shernoff 2012; Wright et al. 2011; Diener et al. 2014b), involves family members, focuses on strengths rather than deficits, and provides vocational support during middle childhood and adolescence. These dimensions are discussed in greater detail below.

NeuroVersity provides a student-centered learning approach. Although structure is provided in terms of the activities that occur during each session, students have a great deal of autonomy to work on a project of their own design and creation. They choose what to design, what tools to use, whether and how to collaborate on the project, and receive individualized instruction from the mentor based on their skills and knowledge. The mentor and facilitator frame feedback positively and rely on the students' internal motivation to create a design based on the students' own interests (Dunn et al. 2014). For example, one student was fascinated with sustainability and created a 3D home that had a pond, garden, solar panels, a cistern for water catchment, and other elements that contributed to sustainability. This student was able to share knowledge and visual strengths through his creation in SketchUp. The mentor uses humor and creates an emotionally supportive atmosphere by modeling mistakes and creating an environment in which mistakes are expected and are viewed as opportunities to learn, by providing specific, positive feedback and by accepting all abilities and designs (Mahoney et al. 2005; Ramey and Rose-Krasnor 2012; Shernoff 2012). Students are expected to learn at their own rate and have the freedom to be creative in their designs. The mentor adjusts his teaching for each student based on the student's skill level with SketchUp (Csikzentmihalyi et al. 1993; Diener et al. 2014b; Dunn et al. 2014).

Unlike interventions that focus on remediating deficits, the strengths-based approach in the program emphasizes what the students are able to learn and do (Baron-Cohen et al. 2011; Grandin 2009, 2011; Mottron 2011). The mentor provides scaffolding when students present their designs to the group so that each student is able to demonstrate their skills and knowledge. The models are a catalyst for sharing SketchUp tools and techniques that each student learns. The presentations accommodate varying levels of verbal skills because of the visual model that can be shared. The mentor also points out the students' successes during the presentations. For example, during a workshop in Salt Lake City, the mentor complimented, "I just want to point out that Kevin (name changed) learned a new tool… Kevin found a new tool, and I am really proud of him. That is really cool." The mentor's ability to highlight and frame the students' skills positively enables the focus to be on what the student is able to achieve, rather than on remediating deficits in skills.

The third component of the program that makes the program special is the central role that families play in the program and the use of a community-based research approach (Wright et al. 2011, 2014). The community-based participatory research model involves parents and community members in the research process and integrates feedback from parents, students, and other family members. They act as co-advisors, as parents have helped determine the structure of the workshops and the research questions addressed and provided input on the data analysis and results. They have helped shape the direction in which the program has gone by providing input on the importance of vocational readiness at earlier ages. Parents and family members are also encouraged to attend the program each day when the students are presenting their designs. By attending the program, they are able to see their student's design, ask supportive questions, and are often surprised by their child's competence with the program and with presentation skills (Wright et al. 2011). The program focuses on cultivating strengths and special interests as a foundation of vocational exploration prior to the transition to adulthood.

The funding of this program has also been quite innovative. The Utah Governor's Office of Economic Development (2014) founded the pilot project for the NeuroVersity students to work on creating 3D designs for a real business, as a transition to real employment. Trimble funded the replication of the workshop program in Boulder, CO, in 2014, and a Google Community Grant funded the replication of the program in The Dalles, Oregon. The University of Central Florida funded the program in Orlando, FL. The Utah Autism Foundation funded the development of the NeuroVersity Curriculum manual, as well as other manuals. Foundation funding (from the McCarthey Foundation) funded laptops for a mobile computer laboratory, and the Utah Autism Council funded video equipment for the program. Internal grants through the University of Utah provided funding for research evaluation of the workshops. Important community partners have included the Columbus Community Center (CCC), Salt Lake School District, and The Dalles School District. The Lassonde Entrepreneur Center at the University of Utah has been instrumental in helping develop a sustainable business model for the program.

Research Results with NeuroVersity Program

The program began in 2010 and has been replicated in seven summer workshop series in several cities, including Salt Lake City, UT; Boulder, CO; Orlando, FL; and The Dalles, OR. It has served over 60 students ranging from 8 to 23 years of age. Plans are currently under way to expand the program internationally to Cape Town, South Africa.

Data evaluating the program have come from multiple sources, including focus groups, individual interviews, participant video documentaries, surveys, observations, and student video evaluations. The results of these evaluations are described here.

Personal Development. A major finding from the evaluation of the NeuroVersity program is the way in which the program enabled individuals to reframe expectations toward a sense of greater competence. The participants in the program are given an opportunity to develop a sense of accomplishment based on the competence that they develop with SketchUp Make (Wright et al. 2011, 2012). Focus groups, parent interviews, and student reports indicate that students gain confidence and reframe their expectations about what they are able to do by participating in this skill- and strength-based program. For example, one mother described her child's feelings as, "I'm good at this, and this is cool that I am good at something! Wahoo! I am finally good at something! Am I like the coolest guy in the whole world?" Parents reported that their children had previously experienced failures in a range of extracurricular activities, yet this program was intrinsically motivating, and thus promoted greater success, leading to true skills and competence over time (Wright et al. 2011). With that competence came a sense of self-efficacy that the youth themselves were able to problem solve, be creative, and learn specific skills. Furthermore, because the program involved family members, who witnessed the development of competence, parents and siblings were also able to change their perceptions of the student with ASD (Diener et al. 2014a; Wright et al. 2011). Grandparents perceived that the program gave them hope for future educational and employment opportunities for their grandchildren (D'Astous et al. 2014; Wright et al. 2012).

The program encourages the development and expression of creativity in that there is not a specific design that the students are required to produce as they are learning the SketchUp program. The students are encouraged to create a design of their own invention. Our Google collaborators provided feedback on the creativity of the models and helped with the development of a creativity assessment for the program (Diener et al. 2014c). This type of creativity is real world and capitalizes on the strengths and interests of youth with ASD. Software development, medical equipment, and engineering advancements are just a few examples that rely on creative applications of technology.

Social Engagement. Although the initial focus of the program was vocational in nature, parents were struck by the spontaneous social engagement that occurred in the program (Wright et al. 2011). Despite parents' fears to the contrary, students rarely sat at their computers without engaging other students. Videotaped observational data indicate that social engagement was non-prompted and unscripted, and occurred with peer and mentor support around common interests (Diener et al. 2014b). Student and parent reports also corroborate the observational findings. For example, a student in Boulder, CO, during the summer of 2014 indicated that his favorite part of the workshops was "the social aspect of it. I enjoy talking with people who see the world like I do." These results extend research from adults with ASD to the way that social supports can be provided to promote social engagement (Muller et al. 2008). Importantly, the most common external support identified in previous research by those with ASD is the opportunity to participate in activities involving shared interests and joint focus. These type of activities, especially when structured in small groups and dyads, create opportunities for membership in a group and provide a sense of belonging (Muller et al. 2008).

The components of the program that may have made it successful in terms of promoting social engagement include purposeful action that provided a challenge to learn real-world skills, and an activity that was intrinsically motivating and enabled the youth to have control over their projects as well as over the timing, extent, and initiation of social engagement (Larson 2000; Ramey and Rose-Krasnor 2012). The components of the program also fit well with most of the components of Lerner's definition of positive youth development, which involves five Cs: competence, caring, connection, character, and confidence (Lerner et al. 2000). The present program involved the development of competence through skills and problem solving as youth work on their 3D designs; caring was modeled and promoted by the adult mentor and facilitators; connection or relationships were developed and supported with peers, mentors, and family members. The program promoted confidence, as described above. Although the program did not include character or morality explicitly, the program did promote the value of treating everyone with respect. Lerner (2004) proposed that ideal youth programs emphasize life skills; provide opportunities for participation and leadership in family, school, and community; and support positive adult–youth relationships. The youth in the present study were motivated to learn software skills that enabled them to impress their peers in the workshops during the presentations. They also used humor to engage their peers during their presentations (Diener et al. 2014b). The students in the program shared common interests in the SketchUp program and used these interests as the foci for social engagement with their peers and with the adult mentor. One student in Boulder, CO, explained it this way: "I like to explain to people how I design things, so that they can learn to do it."

Siblings have also attended the program to watch the presentations with other family members. Interviews with mothers and siblings who observed their brothers' presentations indicate that seeing their brother demonstrating SketchUp skills provided an opportunity for siblings to view their brother positively (Diener et al. 2014a). Sisters reported pride in their brothers' skills, and mothers reported that the sibling pairs engaged one another around SketchUp outside of the workshops. Thus, strength-based programs that include siblings may benefit not only the student with ASD, but also the extended family (Gardiner and Iarocci 2012; Turnbull et al. 2011). A family systems approach suggests that strength-based programming can be most effective if it involves family members.

The program facilitated communication with other grandparents, with their adult children, and with their grandchildren with ASD (Wright et al. 2012). The program gave them a common ground around which to engage other grandparents who also had a grandchild on the spectrum, an opportunity to engage their grandchildren positively, and in some cases strengthened their relationship with their adult children.

Vocational Exploration. The program provides students with an opportunity to explore vocational interests in a technology-focused field. The SketchUp mentor also models an example of a career based on SketchUp skills. The most recent workshop held in Salt Lake City not just provided an opportunity to develop SketchUp skills and explore a technological vocation, but it also provided a partnership with Big D Construction in Utah. The workshops were held at the Salt Lake School District, CCC, a program that finds employment for individuals with disabilities. In the first week of the program, the students followed the curriculum described above for a typical workshop. In the second week, once they had learned the SketchUp skills necessary to complete a 3D design, they were given a job from Big D Construction to generate 3D models using SketchUp from existing two-dimensional building plans. All students were able to complete this directed task, and a review by the building information modeling (BIM) manager at Big D Construction confirmed the accuracy and utility of the models created. Students were paid $50 for completion of the contract job. A student in the summer 2014 Salt Lake City program remarked, "I just like that it's sort of real world so we get some experience on what we would do if we were to join a company like that." Future development includes internship positions for people with ASD with Trimble, the company that owns SketchUp.

Challenges Faced by Program

Despite these successes, the program has faced a number of challenges. As with any community partnership, it has taken substantial time and effort to identify key players, build relationships, and build a team in the community, rather than relying on a single primary community contact. This approach requires additional persistence and energy as well as strong coordination among team members to ensure communication and relationship building. Some potential community partners have left their positions or had insufficient time to devote to the partnership, resulting in dead ends and time invested that did not result in a workshop or partnership. Moreover, despite the innovative funding strategies, it is challenging to obtain funding for sustaining the program. Another challenge has been developing a team of student-centered instructors, because SketchUp experts may not have training or skills in working with youth or working with individuals on the autism spectrum. Thus, training support and ongoing evaluation is critical, and maintaining fidelity and quality controls are essential. We are currently developing a curriculum manual and checklists to ensure high-quality programs at replication sites. Furthermore, small groups of students are necessary to ensure success of the program. Thus, although many parents and students want to participate in the program, demand exceeds capacity and fewer students can be served by the program at this time than desire to participate. Another challenge has been to help parents understand how they can be supportive without being directive. As a result, we are also in the process of creating a parent manual to help guide and inform the parents of youth who participate in the program. Finally, transportation of youth to the program is an issue. Because the program is a half day during the summer, and an after-school program during the fall and spring, it is necessary for youth to have transportation to and from the program during typical business hours. This can prohibit some families from having their student participate in the program. We have had grandparents and other support individuals provide transportation and participate in the family component.

Future Directions

We have a number of directions to pursue in future research. We are interested in the better understanding of individual differences in program effects. For example, what characteristics predict differences in the youths' abilities to complete independent projects on their own for a job site, and what structures and supports need to be provided for success at a job site? Our research indicates that these students are often motivated by the social dimensions of the program, and we need to explore how to incorporate these social dimensions into a job or internship program. We are also interested in better understanding the relative balance between peer and adult led activities as a critical dimension of the program.

Future research will also examine whether authentic language measures during the course of the program demonstrate greater language skills than students demonstrate on standardized language assessments. Preliminary evidence suggests that the interest-based nature of the program may elicit greater language production than students provide in contexts in which they are less engaged or interested. For example, a parent from the Orlando, FL site during Summer 2013 described how her daughter's excitement over learning the SketchUp program motivated her daughter to talk more to family members than she typically did around everyday events: "She was on Skype last night doing crosswords with her twin brother—who is right now overseas—and she told him all about the house she was 'designing with walls, ceiling, kitchen, living room and dining room...' It is rare for her to say several phrases in one conversation!" The student's interest in the program provided an opportunity to engage verbally with her family members.

In summary, technology is an avenue not only for interventions, but also for supporting positive youth development by building on interests and strengths. NeuroVersity is an interest-focused, strength-based, and family-centered technology education program that values neurodiversity and provides youth with opportunities to realize their full potential across the course of life. Our program is unique because it focuses on cultivating and building on strengths and special interests for youth with ASD, not as young children, but as part of their transition to adulthood. Our research demonstrates that the NeuroVersity program impacts (1) Personal Mastery—the program increases participants' self-confidence and self-efficacy as a result of demonstrating 3D technology talents and skills; (2) Social Engagement—program participants engage with peers, family members, and the community by sharing interests and technology talents; (3) Vocational–Technical Training—students develop technology-related job skills associated with Trimble SketchUp. The long-term goal is to build a foundation of computer skills in youth with ASD that match the employment sector that is seeking skilled workers in the technology industry in internships and jobs.

References

Baron-Cohen, S. (2006). Two new theories of autism: Hyper-systemising and assortative mating. *Archives of Disease in Childhood, 91*(1), 2–5. doi:10.1136/adc.2005.075846.

Baron-Cohen, S., Ashwin, E., Ashwin, C., Tavassoli, T., & Chakrabarti, B. (2009). Talent in autism: Hyper-systemizing, hyper-attention to detail and sensory hypersensitivity. *Philosophical Transactions of the Royal Society, 364*, 1377–1383. doi:10.1098/rstb.2008.0337.

Baron-Cohen, S., Ashwin, E., Ashwin, C., Tavassoli, T., & Chakrabarti, B. (2011). The paradox of autism: Why does disability sometimes give rise to talent? In N. Kapur (Ed.), *The Paradoxical Brain* (pp. 274–288). New York: Cambridge University Press.

Baron-Cohen, S., Wheelwright, S., Burtenshaw, A., & Hobson, E. (2007). Mathematical talent is linked to autism. *Human Nature, 18*, 125–141. doi:10.1007/s12110-007-9014-0.

Benson, P. I., Scales, P. C., Hamilton, S. H., & Sesma, A. (2006). Positive youth development: Theory, research, and applications. In W. Damon & R. M. Lerner (Series Eds.), R. M. Lerner (Vol. Ed.), *Handbook of child psychology, Vol. 1: Theoretical models of human development* (6th ed., pp. 894–941). Hoboken, NJ: Wiley

Bernard-Opitz, V., Sriram, N., & Nakhoda-Sapuan, S. (2001). Enhancing social problem solving in children with autism and normal children through computer-assisted instruction. *Journal of Autism and Developmental Disorders, 31*, 377–398. doi:10.1023/A:1010660502130.

Bosseler, A., & Massaro, D. W. (2003). Development and evaluation of a computer-animated tutor for vocabulary and language learning in children with autism. *Journal of Autism and Developmental Disorders, 33*(6), 653–672.

Buggey, T. (2005). Video self-modeling applications with students with autism spectrum disorder in a small private school setting. *Focus on Autism and Other Developmental Disabilities, 20,* 52–63.

Caldwell-Harris, C. L., & Jordan, C. J. (2014). Systemizing and special interests: Characterizing the continuum from neurotypical to autism spectrum disorder. *Learning and Individual Differences, 29,* 98–105. doi:10.1016/j.lindif.2013.10.005.

Cardon, T. (2013). Video modeling imitation training to support gestural imitation acquisition in young children with autism spectrum disorder. *Speech, Language, and Hearing, 16,* 227–238.

Cardon, T., & Wilcox, J. (2011). Promoting imitation in young children with autism: A comparison of reciprocal imitation training and video modeling. *Journal of Autism and Developmental Disorders, 41,* 654–666. doi:10.1007/s10803-010-1086-8.

Caron, M. J., Mottron, L., Rainville, C., & Chouinard, S. (2004). Do high functioning persons with autism present superior spatial abilities? *Neuropsychologia, 42*(4), 467–481.

Charlop-Christy, M. J., & Daneshvar, S. (2003). Using video modeling to teach perspective taking to children with autism. *Journal of Positive Behavior Interventions, 5,* 12–21. doi:10.1177/10983007030050010101.

Chen, X., & Weko, T. (2009). Students who study science, technology, engineering, and mathematics (STEM) in postsecondary education. US Department of Education. NCES #2009-161. Retrieved May 5, 2014 from http://nces.ed.gov/pubsearch/pubsinfo.asp?pubid=2009161

Csikszentimihaly, M., Rathunde, K., & Whalen, S. (1993). *Talented teenagers: The roots of success and failure.* Cambridge, England: Cambridge University Press.

D'Astous, V. A., Wright, S. D., Wright, C. A., & Diener, M. L. (2014). Grandparents of grandchildren with autism spectrum disorders: Influences of engagement. *Journal of Intergenerational Relationships, 11,* 134–147. doi:10.1080/15350770.2013.782744.

Dawes N. P., & Larson, R. (2011). How youth get engaged: Grounded-theory research on motivational development in organized youth programs. *Developmental Psychology, 47,* 259–269. doi:10.1037/a0020729

Dawson, G., & Bernier, R. (2013). A quarter century of progress on the early detection and treatment of autism spectrum disorder. *Developmental and Psychopathology, 25,* 1455–1472. doi:10.1017/S0954579413000710.

Diener, M. L., Anderson, L. L., Wright, C. A., & Dunn, L. (2014a). Sibling relationships of children with autism spectrum disorder in the context of everyday life and a strength-based program. *Journal of Child and Family Studies, 23,* 1–13. doi:10.1007/s10826-014-9915-6.

Diener, M. L., Dunn, L., Wright, C., Wright, D. S., Anderson, L. L., & Smith, K. N. (2014b, in press). A Creative 3D Design Program: Building on interests and social engagement for students with autism spectrum disorder (ASD). *Journal of Disability, Development and Education.*

Diener, M. L., Wright, C. A., Smith, K. N., & Wright, S. D. (2014c). An assessment of visual-spatial creativity in youth with autism spectrum disorder. *Creativity Research Journal, 26,* 328–337. doi:10.1080/10400419.2014.929421.

Donovan, J., & Zucker, C. (2010, Aug 30). Autism's first child. *The Atlantic Monthly, 306,* 78.

Dunn, L., Diener, M. L., Wright, C. A., & Wright, S. D. (2014). The social ecology of vocational readiness in an extracurricular technology program for students with autism. Manuscript under review.

Gardiner, E., & Iarocci, G. (2012). Unhappy (and happy) in their own way: A developmental psychopathology perspective on quality of life for families living with developmental disability with and without autism. *Research in Developmental Disabilities, 33,* 2177–2192. doi:10.1016/j.ridd.2012.06.014.

Golan, O., Ashwin, E., Granader, Y., McClintock, S., Day, K., Leggett, V., & Baron-Cohen, S. (2010). Enhancing emotion recognition in children with autism spectrum conditions: An intervention using animated vehicles with real emotional faces. *Journal of Autism and Developmental Disorders, 40,* 269–279.

Gonzalez, C., Martin, J. M., Minshew, N. J., & Behrmann, M. (2013). Practice makes improvement: How adults with autism out-perform others in a naturalistic visual search task. *Journal of Autism and Developmental Disorders, 43*, 2259–2268. doi:10.1007/s10803-013-1772-4.

Grandin, T. (1995). *Thinking in pictures: My life with autism.* New York: Vintage Books.

Grandin, T. (2009). How does visual thinking work in the mind of a person with autism? A personal account. *Philosphical Transactions of the Royal Society, 364*, 1437–1442. doi:10.1098/rstb.2008.0297.

Grandin, T. (2011). Jobs that teach work skills to kids with ASD. *The Autism Asperger's Digest,* (May/June), 18–19.

Grynszpan, O., Martin, J. C., & Nadel, J. (2008). Multimedia interfaces for users with high functioning autism: An empirical investigation. *International Journal of Human-Computer Studies, 66*, 628–639. doi:10.1016/j.ijhcs.2008.04.001.

Hansen, D. M., & Larson, R. W. (2007). Amplifiers of developmental and negative experiences in organized activities: Dosage, motivation, lead roles, and adult-youth ratios. *Journal of Applied Developmental Psychology, 28*, 360–374.

Heiman, M., Nelson, K. E., Tjus, T., & Gildberg, C. (1995). Increasing reading and communication skills in children with autism through an interactive multimedia program. *Journal of Autism and Developmental Disorders, 25*, 459–480. doi:10.1007/BF02178294.

Hidi, S., & Renninger, K. A. (2006). The four-phase model of interest development. *Educational Psychologist, 41*, 111–127. doi:10.1207/s15326985sep4102_4

Hochhauser, M., & Engel-Yeger, B. (2010). Sensory processing abilities and their relation to participation in leisure activities among children with high-functioning autism spectrum disorder (HFASD). *Research in Autism Spectrum Disorders, 4*, 746–754. doi:10.1016/j.rasd.2010.01.015.

Kalb, C. (2009). SketchUp: Why kids with autism love it. *Newsweek.* Retrieved Jan 15, 2009, from http://www.newsweek.com/sketchup-why-kids-autism-love-it-78513

Kaldy, Z., Giserman, I., Carter, A., & Blaser, E. (2013). The mechanisms underlying the ASD advantage in visual search. *Journal of Autism and Developmental Disorders.* doi:10.1007/s10803-013-1957-x.

Kennedy, D. M., & Banks, R. S. (2011). *Bright not broken: Gifted kids, ADHD, and autism.* San Francisco, CA: Joseey-Bass.

Khowaja, K., & Salim, S. (2013). A systematic review of strategies and computer-based intervention (CBI) for reading comprehension of children with autism. *Research in Autism Spectrum Disorders, 7*, 111–1121.

Kientz, J. A., Goodwin, M. S., Hayes, G. R., & Abowd, G. D. (2014). *Interactive technologies for autism.* San Rafael, CA: Morgan & Claypool Publishers.

Knight, V., McKissick, B., & Saunders, A. (2013). A review of technology-based interventions to teach academic skills to students with autism spectrum disorder. *Journal of Autism and Developmental Disorders, 43*, 2628–2648. doi:10.1007/s10803-013-1814-y.

Larson, R. W. (2000). Toward a psychology of positive youth development. *American Psychologist, 55*, 170–183. doi:10.1037/0003-066X.55.1.170.

Lerner, R. M. (2004). *Liberty: Thriving and civic engagement among America's youth.* Thousand Oaks, CA: Sage.

Lerner, R. M., Fisher, C. B., & Weinberg, R. A. (2000). Toward a science for and of the people: Promoting the civil society through the application of developmental science. *Child Development, 71*, 11–20.

Levy, A., & Perry, A. (2011). Outcomes in adolescents and adults with autism: A review of the literature. *Research in Autism Spectrum Disorders, 5*, 1271–1282.

Mahoney, J. L., Larson, R. W., & Eccles, J. S. (Eds.). (2005). *Organized activities as contexts of development: Extracurricular activities, after-school, and community programs.* Mahwah, NJ: Erlbaum.

McDonald, T. A., & Machalicek, W. (2013). Systematic review of intervention research with adolescents with autism spectrum disorders. *Research in Autism Spectrum Disorders, 6*, 931–938.

Mineo, B. A., Ziegler, W., Gill, S., & Salkin, D. (2009). Engagement with electronic screen media among students with autism spectrum disorders. *Journal of Autism and Developmental Disorders, 39*, 172–187. doi:10.1007/s10803-0080-0616-0.

Moore, M., & Calvert, S. (2000). Brief report: Vocabulary acquisition for children with autism: Teacher or computer instruction. *Journal of Autism and Developmental Disorders, 30*, 359–362.

Mottron, L. (2011). Changing perceptions: The power of autism. *Nature, 479*(7371), 33–35. doi:10.1038/479033a.

Mottron, L., & Belleville, S. (1993). A study of perceptual analysis in a high-level autistic subject with exceptional graphic abilities. *Brain and Cognition, 23*, 279–309.

Muller, E. Schuler, A., Yates, G. B. (2008). Social challenges and supports from the perspective of individuals with Asperger syndrome and other autism spectrum disabilities. *Autism, 12*, 173–190. doi:10.1177/1362361307086664.

Nally, B., Houlton, B., & Ralph, S. (2000). The management of television and video by parents of children with autism. *Autism, 4*, 331–337. doi:10.1177/136261300004003008.

Parsons, S., & Cobb, S. (2011). State-of-the-art virtual reality technologies for children on the autism spectrum. *European Journal of Special Needs Education, 26*, 355–366.

Penngington, R. C. (2010). Computer-assisted instruction for teaching academic skills to students with autism spectrum disorders: A review of the literature. *Focus on Autism and Other Developmental Disabilities, 25*, 239–248. doi:10.1177/1088357610378291.

Ploog, B. O., Scharf, A., Nelson, D., & Brooks, P. J. (2013). Use of computer-assisted technologies (CAT) to enhance social, communicative, and language development in children with autism spectrum disorders. *Journal of Autism and Developmental Disorders, 43*, 301–322. doi:10.1007/s10803-012-1571-3.

Porayska-Pomsta, K., Frauenberger, C., Pain, H., Rajendran, G., Smith, T., Menzies, R., et al. (2012). Developing technology for autism: An interdisciplinary approach. *Personal and Ubiquitous Computing, 16*, 117–127. doi:10.1007/s00779-011-0384-2.

Ramey, H. L., & Rose-Krasnor, L. (2012). Contexts of structured youth activities and positive youth development. *Child Development Perspectives, 6*, 85–91. doi:10.1111/j.1750-8606.2011.00219.x.

Reichow, B. (2012). Overview of meta-analyses on early intensive behavioral intervention for young children with autism spectrum disorders. *Journal of Autism and Developmental Disorders, 42*, 512–520. doi:10.1007/s10803-011-1218-9.

Roskos-Ewoldsen, B., Klinger, L., Klinger, M., Moncrief, A., & Klein, C. (2008). *Creative processes and autism spectrum disorder (unpublished thesis)*. Tuscaloosa, AL: University of Alabama Psychology Department.

Schmidt, M., Laffey, J. M., Schmidt, C. T., Wang, X., & Stichter, J. (2012). Developing methods for understanding social behavior in a 3D virtual learning environment. *Computers in Human Behavior, 28*, 405–413. doi:10.1016/j.chb.2011.10.011.

Selfe, N. (1983). *Normal and anomalous representational drawing ability in children*. London, UK: Metheun.

Shane, H., C., & Albert, P. D. (2008). Electronic screen media for persons with autism spectrum disorders: Results of a survey. *Journal of Autism and Developmental Disorders, 38*, 1499–1508.

Shernoff, D. J. (2012). Engagement and positive youth development: Creating optimal learning environments. In K. R. Harris, S. Graham, & T. Urdan (Eds.), *APA educational psychology handbook: Vol. 2. Individual differences and cultural and contextual factors*. doi:10.1037/13274-008

Shipley-Benamou, R., Lutzker, J. R., & Taubman, M. (2002). Teaching daily living skills to children with autism through instructional video modeling. *Journal of Positive Behavior Interventions, 4*, 165–175. doi:10.1177/10983007020040030501.

Speck, A. A., & Velderman, E. (2013). Examining the relationship between autism spectrum disorders and technical professions in high functioning adults. *Research in Autism Spectrum Disorders, 7*, 606–612.

Taylor, J. L., McPhetters, M., Sathe, N., Dove, D., Veenstra-VanderWeele, J., & Warren, W. (2012). A systematic review of vocational interventions for young adults with autism spectrum disorders. *Pediatrics, 130*, 531–538. doi:10.1542/peds.2012-0682.

Taylor, J. L., & Seltzer, M. M. (2011). Employment and post-secondary educational activities for young adults with autism spectrum disorders during the transition to adulthood. *Journal of Autism and Developmental Disorders, 41*(5), 566–574.

Turnbull, A., Turnbull, H. R., Erwin, E. J., Soodak, L. C., & Shogren, K. A. (2011). *Families, professionals, and exceptionality: Positive outcomes through partnerships and trust* (6th ed.). Columbus, OH: Merrill.

Wagner, M., Cadwallader, T. W., Newman, L., Garza, N., & Blackorby, J. (2002). *The other 80 % of their time: The experiences of elementary and middle school students with disabilities in their non-school hours.* Menlo Park, CA: SRI International. Retrieved August 28, 2014 from http://www.seels.net/designdocs/Wave_1_components_1-7.pdf

Wainer, A. L., & Ingersoll, B. R. (2011). The use of innovative computer technology for teaching social communication to individuals with autism spectrum disorders. *Research in Autism Spectrum Disorders, 5*, 96–107. doi:10.1016/j.rasd.2010.08.002.

Wei, X., Christiano, E., Yu, J., Blackorby, J., Shattuck, P., & Newman, L. (2014a). Postsecondary pathways and persistence for STEM versus non-STEM majors among college students with an autism spectrum disorder. *Journal of Autism and Developmental Disorders, 44*, 1159–1167. doi:10.1007/s10803-013-1978-5.

Wei, X., Wagner, M., Hudson, L., Yu, J. W., & Shattuck, P. (2014b). *Transition to adulthood: Employment, education, and disengagement in individuals with autism spectrum disorders.* Emerging Adulthood: Advance online publication. doi:10.1177/2167696814534417.

Wei, X., Yu, J. W., Shattuck, P., McCracken, M., & Blackorby, J. (2013). Science, technology, engineering, and mathematics (STEM) participation among college students with an autism spectrum disorder. *Journal of Autism and Developmental Disorders, 43*, 1539–1546. doi:10.1007/s10803-012-1700.

Wright, S. D., D'Astous, V., Wright, C. A., & Diener, M. L. (2012). Grandparents of grandchildren with autism spectrum disorder (ASD): Strengthening relationships through technology. *The International Journal of Aging and Human Development, 75*(2), 169–183.

Wright, C. A., Diener, M. L., Dunn, L., Wright, S. D., Linnell, L., Newbold, K., et al. (2011). SketchUp: A technology tool to facilitate intergenerational family relationships for children with autism spectrum disorders (ASD). *Family and Consumer Studies Research Journal, 40*, 136–149. doi:10.1111/j.1552-3934.2011.01200.x.

Wright, C. A., Wright, S. D., Diener, M. L., & Eaton, J. (2014). Autism spectrum disorder and the applied collaborative approach: A review of community-based participatory research and participatory action research. *Journal of Autism, 1*. Retrieved from http://www.hoajonline.com/autism/2054-992X/1/1. doi:10.7243/2054-992X-1-1.

Chapter 10
Evidence-Based Instruction for Students with Autism Spectrum Disorder: TeachTown *Basics*

Phyllis Jones, Catherine Wilcox and Jodie Simon

Introduction

This chapter explores the nature and role of evidence-based practices (EBP) in educational and therapeutic interventions for learners with autism spectrum disorder (ASD). The chapter begins by tracing the historical understandings of autism spectrum disorder (ASD) to the early twentieth century and the shifts that have occurred from psychiatric frames of understanding to current constructions of levels of support, as represented in the DSM-5, required for learners with ASD. The nature and role of EBPs and their evolution in developing interventions for learners with ASD is presented. This is followed by an analysis of an exemplar computer-based program, TeachTown *Basics*, designed specifically for learners with ASD, but which has also been applied to students with other learning issues (for example, intellectual disability). TeachTown *Basics* is a comprehensive intervention program that integrates specific elements of applied behavior analysis (ABA). These ABA elements are detailed before the program is presented. The chapter progresses to an analysis of TeachTown *Basics* in practice. The first part of this section illustrates how three learners with ASD engage with the program at different levels, and the second part of the section discusses school student engagement and progress data gathered through the program. The chapter ends with a discussion of emerging

P. Jones (✉) · C. Wilcox
University of South Florida, Tampa, FL, USA
e-mail: PJones7@usf.edu

C. Wilcox
e-mail: cwilcox3@mail.usf.edu

J. Simon
A Division of Jigsaw Learning, LLC, Teachtown, Woburn, MA, USA
e-mail: jsimon@jigsawlearning.com

© Springer International Publishing Switzerland 2016
T.A. Cardon (ed.), *Technology and the Treatment of Children with Autism Spectrum Disorder*, Autism and Child Psychopathology Series, DOI 10.1007/978-3-319-20872-5_10

research data about the program across a school district, which illustrates the need to engage in further research that builds insight into the experience of students, teachers, and their families who have engaged with TeachTown *Basics*.

Learners with Autism Spectrum Disorder

Leo Kanner first diagnosed autism in the USA in 1943 to describe a group of children with emotional and social problems (Kanner 1943), but it was used earlier in 1911 by a Swiss psychiatrist, Eugen Bleuler, to describe a patient with schizophrenia. At the same time Leo Kanner was working at John Hopkins in the USA, a scientist in Germany, Hans Asperger, identified a similar condition referred to as Asperger's syndrome. The quest to understand and respond to the disorder has received constant but varied attention in the subsequent years. The initial connection to psychiatric frames of understanding and treatment became an established and accepted way of responding to children with autism. During the sixties, the medical profession focused on medications, electric shock therapy, and behavioral change techniques as established treatments. A shift came during the eighties and nineties when sophisticated behavioral therapies and controlled learning environments became a focus of intervention. This shift formed the foundation of the current emphasis on EBPs in 2013 (Wong et al. 2013). Evidence-based strategy can be defined as an instructional strategy, intervention, or teaching program that has resulted in consistent positive results (Simpson 2005).

It is acknowledged that children with ASD are a heterogeneous group, with children and adults displaying different profiles, thus supporting the notion of a spectrum (Lord et al. 2013). The term autism spectrum disorder is used in the DSM-5 (American Psychiatric Association [APA] 2013) to represent children and adults who have both deficits in social communication and social interaction and restricted, repetitive behaviors, interests, and activities. Both components are required for diagnosis of ASD; if there are no restricted and repetitive behaviors, then social communication disorder is diagnosed (APA 2013). The term "spectrum" is adopted to represent a continuum of severity and impact of autism; this occurs in relation to social communication and repetitive behaviors. Some children and adults will fall along the spectrum of severity and this may be compounded by context. In the DSM-5, an ASD diagnosis can be accompanied by a statement of one of three levels of support, which is intended to recognize the severity of the ASD. These levels of support are explained in Table 10.1, ASD Levels of Support.

Evidence-Based Practices

Evidence-based practices (EBPs) have become a marked element of educational and therapeutic approaches to teaching and learning for students with ASD. The movement was captured and crystalized by the National Autism Center (National Autism

Table 10.1 ASD levels of support

Severity level	Social communication	Restricted interests and repetitive behaviors
Level 1 "requiring support"	Issues in social communication cause noticeable impairments. Has difficulty initiating social interactions and demonstrates clear examples of atypical or unsuccessful responses to social overtures of others. May appear to have decreased interest in social interactions	Rituals and repetitive behaviors (RRB's) cause significant interference with functioning in one or more contexts. Resists attempts by others to interrupt RRB's or to be redirected from fixated interest
Level 2 "Requiring substantial support"	Marked issues in verbal and nonverbal social communication skills; social impairments apparent even with Level 1 supports in place; limited initiation of social interactions and reduced or abnormal response to social overtures from others	RRBs and/or preoccupations or fixated interests appear frequently enough to be obvious to the casual observer and interfere with functioning in a variety of contexts. Distress or frustration is apparent when RRB's are interrupted; difficult to redirect from fixated interest
Level 3 "requiring very substantial support"	Severe issues in verbal and nonverbal social communication skills cause severe impairments in functioning; very limited initiation of social interactions and minimal response to social approaches from others	Preoccupations, fixated rituals, and/or repetitive behaviors markedly interfere with functioning in all spheres. Marked distress when rituals or routines are interrupted; very difficult to redirect from fixated interest or returns to it quickly

Center [NAC] 2009) which carried out the first major review of evidence-based research in the field of autism that laid the foundation for the current emphasis on EBP. A research group at the National Autism Center completed a systematic review of the educational and behavioral treatment literature that focused upon the core characteristics of ASD; this literature was published between 1957 and the fall of 2007. The National Autism Center published the National Standards Report (2009) that detailed interventions that fell into groups of established, emerging, unestablished, and ineffective or hurtful. Interventions in the established group include those with sufficient "evidence" available to confidently determine that an intervention produces beneficial effects for individuals on the autism spectrum. That is, these practices are established as effective. Interventions in the emerging group include research on practices that although one or more studies suggest there is a beneficial intervention effect for individuals with ASD, additional high-quality studies are needed to confirm the consistency of the outcome. The unestablished group includes those strategies where little or no evidence exist in order to draw firm conclusions about the intervention's effectiveness with individuals with ASD. The ineffective/

Table 10.2 Established, emerging, and unestablished interventions

Established	Emerging	Unestablished
Antecedent package	Augmentative and alternative communication device	Academic interventions auditory integration training
Behavioral package	Cognitive behavioral intervention package	Facilitated communication Gluten- and Casein-free diet
Comprehensive behavioral treatment for young children	Developmental relationship-based treatment	Sensory integrative package
Joint attention intervention	Exercise	
Modeling	Exposure package	
Naturalistic teaching strategies	Imitation-based interaction	
Peer training package	Initiation training	
Pivotal response training	Language training (production)	
Schedules	Language training (production and understanding)	
Self-management	Massage/touch therapy	
Story-based intervention package		

harmful group was intended to include interventions with several high-quality studies that showed the intervention to be ineffective or harmful. However, there were no interventions included in the ineffective/harmful group. Table 10.2 Established, Emerging, and Unestablished Interventions illustrates the strategies in each group of the National Standards Report.

The review included quantitative research data sets (including experimental group, quasi-experimental group, and single-case designs) and did not include qualitative studies. The EBPs highlighted in the National Standards Report have rapidly become foundational criteria for federal funding of teacher education proposals and an established element of interventions for students with ASD.

Wong et al. carried out a follow-up systematic review of research in 2013 with the purpose of developing a report "that describes a process for the identification of EBPs and also to delineate practices that have sufficient empirical support to be termed evidence-based" (Wong et al. 2013, p. 7). The 2013 review, similar to the earlier review, includes research applicable to implementation in school or community early intervention systems, or home-, hospital-, and community-based

Table 10.3 Nature of learner outcomes across 27 evidence-based strategies

Social	School-readiness skills
Communication	Pre-academic skills
Challenging behavior	Motor
Joint attention	Adaptive/self help
Play	Vocational
Cognitive	Mental health

programs. However, unlike the National Standards Report, it also included research on a number of studies in which the participant had additional learning issues (for example, intellectual and social-emotional). It wanted to address the issue that many traditional systematic review processes have excluded single-case design studies. The report highlighted two broad classes of interventions and identified them as comprehensive treatment models and focused intervention practices (Smith 2013). Comprehensive treatment models include practices designed to achieve a broad learning or developmental impact on the core issues of ASD. Focused interventions are designed to address a single skill or goal of a student with ASD. They address specific learner outcomes and tend to occur over a shorter time period than interventions associated with the comprehensive treatment models. Wong et al. (2013) recognize the symbiotic relationship between focused and comprehensive treatment interventions and highlight the point that they could even occur together; for example, peer-mediated instruction and the LEAP model. The 2013 review incorporated the intervention literature from the years subsequent to the National Standards Report (NAC 2009) initial review (i.e., 2007–2011). 29,105 published research articles were gathered relating to the broad areas of ASD and intervention and this was reduced to 456 with the application of inclusion criteria. Of the 456 studies that were included in the systematic review, 48 utilized a group design, but the majority of studies implemented a single-case design methodology (408). Twenty-seven evidence-based strategies emerged from this meta-analysis that covered a broad range of learner outcomes, as illustrated in Table 10.3: Nature of Learner Outcomes Across 27 Evidence-Based Strategies.

Table 10.4 lists the twenty-seven evidence-based strategies identified by Wong et al. (2013).

The intensive nature of evidence-based autism intervention, which relies heavily on one-to-one intervention, has caused many schools to turn to the growing number of computer-assisted interventions designed specifically for children with ASD.

Technology-Aided Instruction and Intervention (TAII)

Technology-aided instruction and intervention (TAII) is an evidence-based practice that is becoming increasingly popular (US Department of Education 2005). TAII meets evidence-based criteria with nine group design and 11 single-case design

Table 10.4 Twenty-seven evidence-based strategies

Antecedent-based intervention (ABI)	Parent-implemented intervention (PII)
Cognitive behavioral intervention (CBI)	Peer-mediated instruction and intervention (PMII)
Differential reinforcement of alternative, incompatible, or other behavior (DRA/I/O)	Pivotal response training (PRT)
Extinction (EXT)	Prompting (PP)
Functional behavior assessment (FBA)	Reinforcement (R+)
Functional communication training (FCT)	Scripting (SC)
Response interruption/redirection (RIR)	Social narratives (SN)
Self-management (SM)	Social skills training (SST)
Discrete trial teaching (DTT)	Structured play group (SPG)
Exercise (ECE)	Task analysis (TA)
Modeling (MD)	Technology-aided instruction and intervention (TAII)
Naturalistic intervention (NI)	Time delay (TD)
	Video modeling (VM)
	Visual support (VS)

studies. The definition of technology interventions adopted for the meta-analysis included categories of computer-aided instruction and speech-generating devices/VOCA. In addition, different uses of different technology are also represented, including use of smart phones and tablet technology (Wong et al. 2013). TAII includes a group of interventions to address social, communication, behavior, joint attention, cognitive, school-readiness, academic, motor, adaptive, and vocational skills (Odom 2013). Indeed, students with ASD have shown positive gains using TAII (Hetzroni and Shalem 2005; Massaro and Bosseler 2006). Advantages of TAII include increased learning following consistency of a clearly defined task, reduced distractions leading to more focus of attention (Murray 1997), and supporting the ability to initiate, maintain, or terminate a behavior (Goldsmith and LeBlanc 2004). There are a number of TAII programs designed specifically for students with ASD that

- Teach the recognition of faces and emotions (Bölte et al. 2002; Faja et al. 2008; Silver and Oakes 2001);
- Develop spatial planning (Grynszpan et al. 2007);
- Teach functional activities of daily living, safety skills (Josman et al. 2008);
- Develop vocabulary (Massaro and Bosseler 2006);
- Develop reading skills (Ramdoss et al. 2011);
- Improve vocal imitation (Bölte et al. 2010); and
- Develop social participation skills (Parsons and Mitchell 2002).

Discrete Trial Training (DTT)

Discrete trial training (DTT) is an effective teaching procedure derived from the principles of ABA and is used in teaching skills to students with autism. The primary focus is on skill acquisition when teaching early learning skills by breaking down skills into small, learnable parts appropriate to the developmental level of the child. DTT has four distinct parts: (1) the presentation of a stimulus, (2) the child's response, (3) the consequence, and (4) a short pause between the consequence and the next presentation of stimuli. DTT promotes the development of communication/language, adaptive behavior, cognitive/academic skills, and social skills and reduces interfering behaviors. The structured procedures have been effective in teaching children a predictable process for learning.

Pivotal Response Training (PRT)

Pivotal response training (PRT) is a naturalistic intervention that builds on learner initiative and interests, and supports developing (and increasing) communication skills, developing language, play, and social behaviors. PRT was developed to enhance pivotal learning variables: motivation, responding to multiple cues, self-management, and self-initiations of social interactions (Koegel and Frea 1993; Suhrheinrich et al. 2007). The skills are described as pivotal because they are the foundational skills upon which learners with ASD can make widespread and generalized improvements in many other areas (Suhrheinrich et al. 2007). Some central components of PRT include: child choice, reinforcement of successive attempts, incorporation of maintenance tasks, and direct/natural reinforcers that are contingent on appropriate behavior.

TeachTown *Basics*: An Exemplar Program that Is Informed by Evidence-Based Practices

TeachTown *Basics* is an example of a computer-based (TAII) comprehensive intervention program that has the foundations of ABA. An empirical study of the program, which is described in more detail at the end of this chapter, provided documentation for supporting TAII as an evidence-based practice in the Wong et al. (2013) review. ABA involves constructing intervention strategies that outline the antecedents and consequences, which result in the increase in positive skills (Cooper et al. 2007). Data are collected in order to systematically determine interventions to produce positive outcomes for the individual. The instructional design of TeachTown *Basics* is heavily influenced by methodologies within ABA by integrating two evidenced-based strategies: DTT and PRT.

TeachTown *Basics*: An Overview

TeachTown *Basics* is designed for students' with ASD between the developmental ages of 2–7 years. The program includes more than 500 computer lessons to teach skills across six learning domains: language arts, language development, mathematics, cognitive skills, adaptive skills, and social and emotional skills. It has five levels of instruction to meet the needs of children at different developmental stages up to 12 years of age. The computer lessons offer a focused learning environment where the child works on the computer and completes lessons that incorporate the basic principles of ABA. The computer lessons are matched and aligned with integrated generalization lessons which are conducted in the natural environment and developed from the principles of PRT. The student works on the computer lessons independently and the program self-adjusts according the student's progress. The computer portion of the program does not require external expertise in ABA. A key feature of the program is the ability to select lessons that align to a student's individualized education plan (IEP) goals.

When starting a student on the program, the facilitator completes a student placement questionnaire on the computer that assists in determining the student's level (one through five) across the six learning domains. The student progresses through the curriculum at an individualized pace. In the program, the student is given a pretest before a new skill is introduced. If the student correctly responds (unprompted) to 80 % or higher of the trials within the pretest, the lesson is considered "mastered" and the program automatically advances the student to the next lesson. However, if the student scores less than 80 % correct on the pretest, a series of training exercises follow (with and without prompting). When the student scores 80 % or greater correct on training exercises with no prompting, a posttest is given. If the student passes the posttest (given the 80 % criterion), he or she progresses to the next lesson. A student that fails the posttest repeats the process until achieving 80 % unprompted correct responses on the posttest. Stimuli in tests are different than stimuli in training exercises to facilitate generalization of concepts rather than memorization of specific target stimuli. The program is adaptive and will automatically adjust the curriculum based on student's performance.

During a computer session, a student automatically receives reinforcement for correct responses in the form of 15–45 s of animated reward games delivered on a variable ratio. Administrators have the flexibility to thin the schedule of reinforcement. Correct responses are immediately reinforced with verbal praise and visual graphics. The computer lessons use the discrete trial format with a within-stimulus prompting procedure. Verbal instruction is given to the student to click on the correct response from a field of 3–8 choices. These verbal instructions are presented in a variety of ways to promote generalization. The multiple exemplars of stimuli are used for each concept taught in order to facilitate generalization. As of the date of this chapter, the program includes over 24,000 such exemplars. Multiple concepts (e.g., dog and cat) are taught in the same set of trials and the instructions vary slightly from trial to trial so that the child must listen to the instructions for every trial. If the student begins to answer incorrectly, the program systematically fades out the distracters prompting the student to select the correct response and teaching a child to discriminate between stimuli. As students master lessons within the program, automatic maintenance trials are interspersed with training trials to ensure whether the student maintains the skills learned.

Generalization Lessons

A second component of the program is generalization lessons that are designed for the teacher to provide through direct instruction off the computer. The generalization lessons correspond directly to the on-computer lessons. They are written in a lesson plan format and use the principles of pivotal response training. An illustration of one generalization lesson is shown in Fig. 10.1. The generalization lessons focus on skills not targeted on the computer (e.g., expressive language; imitation, and fine motor skills) and are intended to enhance generalization of skills already learned on the computer into the natural environment of the classroom.

TeachTown in Practice

An automated data collection, tracking, and reporting system assess progress as each student moves through the computer curriculum. This allows school staff to assess the effectiveness of the intervention and to determine which skills may need more targeted work in the natural environment through the generalization lessons. This reporting system enables teachers, parents, and professionals to assess student progress and make evidenced-based decisions for instruction. In addition, reports are available for school administrators to assess student, teacher, and parent usage of the program. A communication system is provided within the software for school staff, parents, and various educational team members to document anecdotal reports, daily information about the student's performance, or any other relevant information to the student's success with the program in order to ensure the entire team is communicating effectively. Internet-based synchronization and real-time updating of data allow the sharing of information across families and other educational team members. This feature allows for the program to be used at home and in other learning environments (e.g., the speech language pathologist's clinic, and day care).

Student Generated Data

A description of the use of TeachTown *Basics* by three first-grade students between September and November 2014 serves to illustrate how the program can respond to individual student strengths and needs. All data have been generated through the

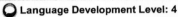 **Coloring Pages**

○ **Language Development Level: 4**

Connection to Computer Curriculum
TeachTown®: Basics MC: Color-Object

Learning Objectives
Your student will request an item of specific color to complete a task.

Related Skills: Expressive language, fine motor, receptive language

 Materials Needed
Coloring pages (such as color-by-number sheets) for each student, markers or crayons

Preparation:
Collect the needed materials in an appropriate area.

 Instructions

1. Tell your students that they are going to color pictures. Pass out a coloring page to each student. Make sure that each coloring page has at least two items on it to color.

2. Color one of the pages yourself and show it to your students as an example. Tell your students, "I need a green marker for the tree." Then, use the green marker. Tell them, "I need a blue marker for the sky", then color the sky.

3. Keep the markers out of your students' reach and ask them to color their pictures Have your students request specific. For example, your student could say, "I need purple."

4. Wait for them to request a specific color marker before handing it to them. (If your student does not make a request, prompt them with subtle hints like, "What do you need?" or with peer modeling, "I like how Sally asked for a blue marker!"

5. Encourage your students to make comments about their colors. Say things like, "Wow, you're coloring a flower purple!"

6. When your students are done, have them share their pictures with the other students.

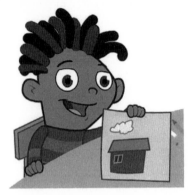

Make It Fun: Find coloring pages of your students' favorite animals or characters.

Make It Meaningful: Talk about the color of certain objects as they work on the activity. For example, "You colored the sky blue, just like our chairs!"

Make It Easy: The students will choose a color from a field of 2 to use to complete a task. For example, hold up two markers and ask, "Do you want to use red or blue?" Have the student reach for or point to the marker they would like to use to color.

Make It Hard: The students will request specific items by color to complete a task. For example, put a container of markers, crayons, and colored pencils, and have the student request a specific item by color, e.g. "I want a blue colored pencil" or "I need a green crayon".

Related Activities:
1. Play a guessing game and use colors to describe the item that you want your students to guess. "I'm thinking of someone who is wearing a green and yellow shirt", etc.

2. On each page of a journal, write a phrase that uses a color to describe something (e.g., red cat, yellow banana, purple flower, etc.). Have your students draw pictures that go with each phrase.

⚊ **TEACHTOWN**: Basics   **(35)**   Appropriate for 🏫 🏠 👥 🧑 School Home Group Individual   Lessons

Language Development – Level: 4

Fig. 10.1 Example of a generalization lesson

program's automatic data collection and reporting system. Student identifiers have been removed to protect anonymity, but permission has been gained from the students' parents to share these data. Three reports are available for the teacher to download about individual students: (a) the *Individual Progress Report* presents lesson content and corresponding off-computer generalization lessons for all lessons worked on by the student as well as performance data on lessons in progress, (b) the *Lesson Progress Graphs* displays in a bar graph the number of trials, level of prompting, and accuracy data for a particular lesson, and (c) the *Average Exercises to Mastery and Gain in Percent Correct for Mastered Lessons Report* displays in a bar graph the distribution of lessons mastered across content domains and the average number of trials taken to master those lessons. The description that follows details information from each of these reports, but due to space, does not replicate the reports per se. The program progresses through five levels of difficulty. As an introduction to the students, Table 10.5 gives an overview of student level at entry and after 12 weeks of program use, as well as number of minutes spent working on lessons in each of the program's six content domains.

Student One

K.A. is a first-grade student identified with ASD with a severity classification of Level 2, "Requiring substantial support." He needs visual supports to increase his communication skills and also needs maximum prompting to interact with peers. K. A. performs below the grade level in all academic areas. Examples of his performance include reading approximately 20 sight words and rote counting to 50. K.A. entered the TeachTown *Basics* curriculum at level 1.0 in all six content domains. Over 12 weeks of using the program, the program adjusted his level according to his performance on the lessons in each domain. By the end of 12 weeks, K.A. had progressed between one-tenth and one-half of a level in four out of six domains (see the top panel of Table 10.5).

Over the 12 weeks, K.A. used the computer program approximately 3 sessions a week for 12 min a session for a total of 7 h. During this time, he worked on 13 lessons. Most lessons target between 2 and 4 concepts. In September, he mastered two lessons where he failed the pretest and then subsequently passed the training exercises and posttest. One lesson mastered was visual perceptual matching of toys (i.e., ball, swing, slide, bubbles, doll, puzzle, book, and teddy bear), and the other was receptively identifying characters from the program, both in the social and emotional domain. In these lessons, it took him on average three training exercises, representing 45 trials, to improve from the failed pretest score to the passed posttest score.

K.A. is currently working on 11 lessons where he failed the pretest and is working on the training exercises or posttest for those lessons. The title of each lesson in progress as well as the date the lesson was last worked on is shown on the *Individual Progress Report*. For K.A., all but two of the lessons in progress have

Table 10.5 Student level in the computer portion of the TeachTown *Basics* curriculum at entry and after 12 weeks of using the program, and time spent working on lessons in each domain

	Adaptive skills	Cognitive skills	Language arts	Language development	Mathematics	Social and emotional
KA						
Level at entry	1.0	1.0	1.0	1.0	1.0	1.0
Level after 12 weeks	1.0	1.1	1.2	1.0	1.5	1.1
LD						
Level at entry	3.0	2.0	1.0	1.0	3.0	1.0
Level after 12 weeks	3.1	2.3	1.4	1.3	3.8	1.7
JL						
Level at entry	3.0	3.0	1.0	2.0	3.0	1.0
Level after 12 weeks	3.0	3.0	2.0	2.4	3.8	2.4

been worked on over the past one to two weeks, including one lesson that is displayed in red indicating that he appears to be struggling and may need additional help in order to master the material. The *Lesson Progress Graph* allows the teacher to pinpoint the content with which K.A. is struggling in this lesson. It shows that K. A. has not mastered receptive identification of toys, ball, and swing, after completing 31 training exercises of which he received prompting in 16. In all, K.A. has spent 64 min or 20 computer sessions working on this task without achieving mastery. The *Lesson Progress Graph* also indicates which generalization lesson the teacher can use to reinforce instruction relating to the skill K.A. is struggling with.

Student Two

L.D. is a first-grade student who has ASD with a severity classification of Level 1, "Requiring support." Severe tantrums have caused significant interference in the classroom, but have improved over time. He is performing close to grade level in all academic areas. L.D. entered the TeachTown program at level 1.0 in the language arts, language development, and social and emotional domains, at level 2.0 in the cognitive skills domain, and at level 3.0 in the mathematics and adaptive skills domains. By the end of 12 weeks, L.D. had shown progress in all six domains, with increases between one-tenth and four-fifths of a level (see the middle panel of Table 10.5).

Over 12 weeks, he used the program on average 4 sessions a week for approximately 13 min per session for a total of 12 h during which he engaged with a total of 31 lessons. Of the 31 lessons worked on, he mastered 7 across all six domains. He had the least difficulty mastering the math lessons of number identification and matching numbers to quantities, and the most difficulty mastering receptive identification of the emotional states scared and sick, and associating cat with mouse, as shown by the number of exercises it took to master the material. L.D. is currently working on 24 lessons. The *Individual Progress Report* identifies one lesson in progress where L.D. appears to be struggling and may need support in order to master the material—the lesson targets identification of the emotions happy, sad, angry, and surprised. Other tasks he appears to be struggling with based on a relatively high number of sessions spent on the material includes identifying mothers and fathers, matching non-exact images of dolphins, whales and fish, and identifying the articles of clothing dress and veil. The *Individual Progress Report* displays the off-computer generalization lesson(s) that coordinates with each of these lessons in progress.

Student Three

J.L. is a first-grade student who has ASD classified by his teacher as Level 1, "Requiring support." Although he enjoys interacting with his peers, he has difficulties with social communication skills. He is easily distracted and interrupts ongoing tasks to attend to noises or events that are usually ignored by others. He performs at grade level in reading and just below grade level in math. In the TeachTown program, J.L. showed progress in four out of the six content domains. He increased from level 1.0 to 2.0 in the language arts domain, 1.0 to 2.4 in the social and emotional domain, 2.0 to 2.4 in the language development domain, and 3.0 to 3.8 in the math domain (see the bottom panel of Table 10.5).

J.L. used the program on average 5 sessions a week for approximately 15 min per session between September and the end of November for a total of 15 h. During this time, he engaged with 24 lessons. Of these 24 lessons, he mastered 15 lessons. The *Average Number of Exercises and Gain in Percent Correct for Mastered Lessons* shows that he mastered lessons across all six content domains and his efficiency at mastering material in these lessons varied across domains. He was least efficient mastering material in the cognitive skills domain, where it took him on average 14 exercises to master a lesson relative to 2–4 exercises in the other domains. The *Lesson Progress Graph* corresponding to the lesson mastered in the cognitive skills domain shows that he had difficulty identifying an animal that was not a tiger or a monkey.

Of the nine lessons he has in progress, three are flagged for needing support. The *Lesson Progress Graphs* that correspond to these lessons reveal that the material J.L. is having difficulty with includes identifying the sounds /ch/ and /d/, identifying tools for measuring weight and length, and identifying whether the number of objects in one group is greater than or less than the number in the other. The *Individual Progress Report* presents the off-computer generalization lessons that coordinate with each of these skill areas.

School-Level Generated Data

There are four types of school-level reports that allow teachers and administrators an overview of how the program is being used in individual classrooms across the whole school. The reports are as follows:

1. *Program Use by Facilitator (Teacher)*
2. *Progress by Student*
3. *Lessons Mastered Relative to Hours of Use Scatterplot*
4. *Average Number of Exercises and Gain in Percent Correct for Mastered Lessons.*

The *Program Use by Facilitator Report* summarizes program usage data for multiple teachers and paraeducators, referred to as facilitators. This report shows for each facilitator the average number of sessions and minutes per week of instruction students working under the facilitator is receiving in the program, and a bar graph meter displays the extent to which students working under that facilitator have used the program. Visually scanning the bar graphs allows an administrator to quickly identify which facilitators are using the program at or above the recommended guidelines.

The *Progress by Student Report* allows administrators an overview of how students are responding to the program. It summarizes progress data as a student moves through the computer curriculum for multiple students. This report allows a teacher or administrator to monitor across students the amount of time spent working on the computer lessons relative to the number of lessons in progress (i.e., lessons where the student failed the pretest and is currently working on the exercises or posttest for that lesson), the number of lessons mastered (i.e., lessons where the student failed the pretest and then subsequently passed the exercises and posttest), and the average number of training exercises needed to move the student from their pretest to their posttest score on mastered lessons. The *Lessons Mastered Relative to Hours of Use Scatterplot Report* displays the relationship between students' total number of hours spent on the program and their total lessons mastered. This helps to visually identify students who are outliers, in particular students who have spent several hours on the program with relatively few lessons mastered. Lastly, the *Average Number of Exercises and Gain in Percent Correct for Mastered Lessons by Domain* allows an overview of the efficiency with which lessons are being mastered in each of the six content domains for all students in a class or school. Efficiency is measured as the average number of training exercises taken to improve from a failed pretest score to a passed posttest score across all lessons mastered.

Emerging Research Data

A study was carried out in four elementary schools in Los Angeles Unified School District (Whalen et al. 2010). The study followed children who were enrolled in a special day class program for students with an eligibility of autism spectrum disorder in four preschool and four *K*-1 classrooms. The ratio of adults to students was 1:2, with no more than eight students in the class. The physical structure of the classroom was based on TEACCH principles and direct instruction utilized an ABA approach. Eight classrooms were randomly assigned to a TeachTown *Basics* intervention or to a no-TeachTown *Basics* comparison group. Teachers in the intervention group received two hours of training. Over a three-month period, TeachTown *Basics* was used with 22 students for 15 min a day on the computer and 20 min a day in the generalization lessons. The study offered comparison data with the 25 children who did not have access to the program.

Baseline data were gathered from all the children in the study using eight language and cognitive skill areas measured by the Brigance Inventory of Early Development (Brigance and Glascoe 2004), a criterion-referenced early development assessment, the Peabody Picture Vocabulary Test (PPVT-3, Dunn and Dunn 1997) and the Expressive Vocabulary Test (EVT; Williams 1997), standardized measures of receptive and expressive language, respectively. At pretest, the intervention and comparison groups were similar in terms of chronological age and also severity of autism characteristics, as measured by the Childhood Autism Rating Scale (CARS, Schopler et al. 1986). Over the three-month period, 15 out of 22 children in the intervention group mastered lessons in TeachTown *Basics*, with an average of 4–5 computer-based lessons mastered over the three-month period. Compared with the 25 students in the comparison group, students in the intervention group showed more improvement on all cognitive and language outcome measures. The intervention preschool group had statistically significantly larger raw score gains (9 pre- to 23 post-intervention) than the comparison preschool group (10 pre- to 15 post-intervention) on the PPVT. All other group differences did not reach statistical significant which may be due to the small sample sizes. The study found a significant positive relationship between the number of TeachTown *Basics* computer-based lessons mastered and pre- to posttest change on the overall Brigance score; that is, children who mastered more lessons showed larger increases in Brigance scores.

The LAUSD study shows the potential promise of the program. It was, however, designed on a small sample size, over a short duration of time, and there was lack of data on relevant variables, thus differences in outcomes between TeachTown and comparison groups may have been due to unmeasured factors and not to the effects of the program. Research published by TeachTown which emerges from data gathered by three additional school districts in independent evaluations (TeachTown 2013) also points to the promising trend of learning gains for students engaged in the program. This too supports the need for further larger scale research on TeachTown *Basics*.

Conclusion

This chapter has discussed the evolving landscape for evidence-based interventions for students with ASD before introducing the reader to TeachTown *Basics,* a computer-based comprehensive intervention program that is founded in ABA. The explicit connections to DTT and PRT have also been highlighted. It has been shown that Teachtown *Basics* is informed by evidence-based intervention strategies (Wong et al. 2013). After describing the TeachTown *Basics* program, a discussion of the role of the built-in student data collection, collation, and analysis followed, giving an insight into how teachers, other professionals and school administrators receive accurate accounts of student engagement in the program. This is offered through vignettes of three first graders and illustrates how individual students engage with the program in personalized and different ways. A brief overview of the LAUSD report (Whalen et al. 2010) closes out the chapter. This research points to the potential of TeachTown *Basics* as a valuable tool in the successful teaching and learning of students with ASD (many of whom have additional learning issues), but also highlights the need for further research. Such research could involve large-scale data sets, single-case design, and also more qualitative projects that build insight into the experience of students, teachers, and their families of engaging with TeachTown *Basics.*

References

American Psychiatric Association. (2013). *Diagnostic and statistical manual of mental disorders* (5th ed.). Washington, DC.: Author.

Bölte, S., Feineis-Matthews, S., Leber, S., et al. (2002). The development and evaluation of a computer-based program to test and to teach the recognition of facial affect. *International Journal of Circumpolar Health, 61*(2), 61–68.

Bölte, S., Golan, O., Goodwin, M. S., & Zwaigenbaum, L. (2010). What can innovative technologies do for autism spectrum disorders? *Autism, 14*(3), 155–159.

Brigance, A.H., & Glascoe, F.P. (2004). *Brigance diagnostic inventory of early development II.* North Billerica, Mass: Curriculum Associates

Cooper, J., Heron, T., & Heward, W. (2007). *Applied behavior analysis* (2nd ed.). Upper Saddle River, NJ: Pearson Prentice Hall.

Dunn, L., & Dunn, L. (1997). *Peabody picture vocabulary test-3rd edition (PPVT-3).* Circle Pines, MN: American Guidance Service.

Faja, S., Aylward, E., Bernier, R., et al. (2008). Becoming a face expert: A computerized face-training program for high-functioning individuals with autism spectrum disorders. *Developmental Neuropsychology, 33*(1), 1–24.

Goldsmith, T. R., & LeBlanc, L. A. (2004). Use of technology in interventions for children with autism. *Journal of Early and Intensive Behavior, 1,* 166–178.

Grynszpan, O., Martin, J., & Nadel, J. (2007). Exploring the influence of task assignment and output modalities on computerized training for autism. *Interaction Studies, 8*(2), 241–266.

Hetzroni, O. E., & Shalem, U. (2005). From logos to orthographic symbols: A multilevel fading computer program for teaching nonverbal children with autism. *Focus on Autism and Other Developmental Disabilities, 20*(4), 201–212.

Josman, N., Ben-Chaim, H., Friedrich, S., et al. (2008). Effectiveness of virtual reality for teaching street-crossing skills to children and adolescents with autism. *International Journal on Disability and Human Development, 7*(1), 49–56.

Kanner, L. (1943). Autistic disturbances of affective contact. *Nervous Child, 2,* 217–250.

Koegel, R. L., & Frea, W. D. (1993). Treatment of social behavior in autism through modification of pivotal social skills. *Journal of Applied Behavior Analysis, 26*(3), 369–377.

Lord, C., Cook, E. H., Leventhal, B. L., & Amaral, D. G. (2013). Autism spectrum disorders. *Autism: The Science of Mental Health, 28,* 217.

Massaro, D. W., & Bosseler, A. (2006). Read my lips: The importance of the face in a computer animated tutor for vocabulary learning by children with autism. *Autism, 10*(5), 495–510.

Murray, D. (1997). Autism and information technology: Therapy with computers. In S. Powell & R. Jordan (Eds.), *Autism and learning: A guide to good practice* (pp. 100–117). London: David Fulton Publishers.

National Autism Center (2009). National standards report. Randolph, MA: Author.

Odom, S. L. (2013). *Technology-aided instruction and intervention (TAII) fact sheet.* Chapel Hill: The University of North Carolina, Frank Porter Graham Child Development Institute. The National Professional Development Center on Autism Spectrum Disorders.

Parsons, S., & Mitchell, P. (2002). The potential of virtual reality in social skills training for people with autistic spectrum disorders. *Journal of Intellectual Disability Research, 46*(5), 430–443.

Ramdoss, S., Mulloy, A., Lang, R. O., Reilly, M., Sigafoos, J., Lancioni, G., et al. (2011). Use of computer-based interventions to improve literacy skills in students with autism spectrum disorders: A systematic review. *Research in Autism Spectrum Disorders, 5,* 1306–1318.

Schopler, E., Reichler, R. J., & Renner, B. R. (1986). The childhood autism rating scale (CARS): For diagnostic screening and classification of autism. New York: Irvington.

Silver, M., & Oakes, P. (2001). Evaluation of a new computer intervention to teach people with autism or asperger syndrome to recognize and predict emotions in others. *Autism: the International Journal of Research and Practice, 5*(3), 299–316.

Simpson, R. (2005). Evidence-based practices and students with autism spectrum disorders. *Focus on Autism and Other Developmental Disabilities, 20*(3), 140–149.

Smith, T. (2013). What is evidence-based behavior analysis? *Behavior Analyst, 36,* 7–33.

Suhrheinrich, J., Stahmer, A., & Schreibman, L. (2007). A preliminary assessment of teachers' implementation of pivotal response training. *Journal of Speech, Language Pathology, and Applied Behavior Analysis, 2,* 8–20.

TeachTown. (2013). *Evidence of effectiveness: Research guide.* Woburn, MA: Author.

Whalen, C., Moss, D., Ilan, A. B., Vaupel, M., Fielding, P., MacDonald, K., et al. (2010). Efficacy of TeachTown: Basics computer-assisted intervention for the intensive comprehensive autism program in Los Angeles unified school district. *Autism, 14*(13), 179–197.

Williams, K. T. (1997). *Expressive vocabulary test (EVT).* Circle Pines, MN: American Guidance Service.

Wong, C., Odom, S. L., Hume, K., Cox, A. W., Fettig, A., Kucharczyk, S., et al. (2013). *Evidence-based practices for children, youth, and young adults with autism spectrum disorder.* Chapel Hill: The University of North Carolina, Frank Porter Graham Child Development Institute, Autism Evidence-Based Practice Review Group.

Chapter 11
Mobile Technology as a Prosthesis: Using Mobile Technology to Support Community Engagement and Independence

Kevin M. Ayres, Sally B. Shepley, Karen H. Douglas, Collin Shepley and Justin D. Lane

Portable computer technology has existed since the late 1960s and early 1970s but was largely restricted to research and development centers (e.g., PARC). In 1989, Apple introduced a portable computer that weighed in at 16 lbs and cost over $6,000. In the late 1990s, researchers began using other mobile technologies such as portable DVD players (Mechling and Stephens 2009) and handheld computers (Davies et al. 2002) as instructional supports for children and adults with ASD and intellectual disability (ID). Broadly speaking, as technology became more mobile and less expensive, researchers found new ways to use these tools for instruction.

To facilitate a quality discussion of mobile technology, however, we must first define what "mobile technology" will encompass for this chapter. Historically speaking, one might argue that books are a mobile technology far more advanced than stone tablets and they are certainly much more portable. The focus of this chapter though will try to move closer to the edges of technological advancement and beyond the technology of a paperback book. Not to oversimplify, but the technology this chapter addresses incorporates some form of computer technology (electronic device designed to store, display, and process data; American Heritage Dictionary 2000) and can in general be carried in one hand or worn on the body.

The ubiquity of mobile technology establishes it as a socially valid tool for teaching and support. Two main principles will moderate this discussion. First and foremost, technology (whether a book or a laptop) is only a tool. Alone, technology cannot truly teach (even with self-instruction, one must learn to self-instruct first);

K.M. Ayres (✉) · S.B. Shepley
The University of Georgia, Athens, GA, USA
e-mail: kayres@uga.edu

K.H. Douglas
Illinois State University, Normal, IL, USA

C. Shepley
Oconee County Schools, Watkinsville, GA, USA

J.D. Lane
The University of Kentucky, Lexington, KY, USA

© Springer International Publishing Switzerland 2016
T.A. Cardon (ed.), *Technology and the Treatment of Children with Autism Spectrum Disorder*, Autism and Child Psychopathology Series, DOI 10.1007/978-3-319-20872-5_11

someone (like a teacher) has to plan for how learning will occur with the technology. Second, computer technology changes very rapidly. Therefore, most of the discussion in this chapter will hinge on the application of the technology for teaching rather than on the specifications of the technology. Discussing the latest mobile phone from Apple (iPhone® 6 at the time of this writing) would only waste space and render large portions of the chapter obsolete less than a year after publication. Instead, if we attend to ways of using technology in general and the evidence base behind it, we can provide educators with a more practical reference.

The final consideration to address before moving forward is a conceptual distinction between instructional technology and assistive technology. This is not a perfect taxonomy as much as a means to help organize the discussion and narrow our focus. As suggested by Ayres et al. (2014), we consider instructional technology a tool (e.g., software) designed to help a learner acquire a set of responses (e.g., multiplication facts), typically used for a short period of time during the acquisition or fluency phase of learning (i.e., the technology will no longer be used once the learner can perform the target behavior independently). In contrast, assistive technology (or supporting technology) refers to tools a user might rely on indefinitely (e.g., an augmentative communication device, a calculator, or text/screen reader). Our focus will remain on the latter, assistive technology, and how this can help support greater independence and integration into the community, but more specifically how the technology can support self-management (SM). In this way, mobile technology can serve as a prosthesis: essentially an external support designed to compensate for something that is missing. Linsley (1964) wrote a pioneering paper in which he stated, "Children are not retarded [sic]. Only their behavior in average environments is sometimes retarded. In fact, it is modern science's ability to design suitable environments for these children that is retarded" (p. 62). He goes on to discuss the idea of learning prosthesis. It seems that modern science may currently be providing quality portable prosthesis that can help individuals better access their environments.

Technology as a Teaching Tool

Though we will not discuss technology as a teacher-directed instructional tool, we want to highlight some brief uses of technology as an aide for instruction. This will help provide some context for later discussion around self-instruction. Examples of technology as an aide for instruction include using (a) an MP3 player and headphones as a prompting device for teaching daily living skills (Taber-Doughty 2005), (b) a portable DVD player to teach cooking tasks (Mechling and Stephens 2009), and (c) handheld computers (early HP windows based and older, now defunct Palm OS) to teach a range of academic and vocational skills (Davies et al. 2002; Mechling and Savidge 2011). What these examples have in common is that a teacher used technology-delivered prompting rather than more traditional teacher-delivered prompting for the learners to acquire the target skills. This advancement in technology-based instruction with mobile devices is laudable as it created opportunities for further development and advancement. This work served as evidence that these tools have value to educators as well as students. In addition, often these materials had practical utility for educators beyond their initial use because they could easily be reused with other learners and provided consistency across instructors (i.e., a teacher and paraprofessional use the same prompt).

Once students acquire new skills like those referenced above, they require less assistance from parents, teachers, or peers in accessing their community. Educators desire outcomes like this because they represent the success of their work. Thinking hypothetically for a moment, how many combinations of skills does a person need to learn in order to live independently in their community? Certainly more than 100, probably more than 1000, and that number will differ from student to student and from location to location. Regardless of whether we settle on an exact number, the figure will surpass what any reasonable educator can hope to accomplish in the approximately 18 years of public schooling a student receives. Whereas students without ASD learn innumerable skills that facilitate independence incidentally through experience and observing others, many children with ASD require direct instruction to acquire the same skills (Wolery and Hemmeter 2011). Given that time constraints in a school setting a teacher cannot feasibly provide direct instruction for all of the skills a student needs to maximize their life outcomes. Just like teachers do not teach children to spell every single word they will ever need to learn, they should not teach children with ASD every skill they will need to learn. Rather they should consider teaching them a means to learn any new skill just as we teach children to identify the letter sounds in the words they want to spell. This is the role technology (i.e., assistive technology) can help fulfill.

Technology as Prosthesis

For technology to serve as a daily (or even intermittent) support, an individual has to learn to use the technology for this purpose. Think of how you learned to search for information online. Likely, you required at least a little initial instruction to input commands and then sift through information. Teaching someone to use technology requires not only the instruction on how to manipulate the technology but also on how to respond to prompts and other supports offered by the technology. Mobile technology offers an almost ideal platform for self-instruction because of its portability and usability. Further, no one standing in the middle of a store or on the street corner looks out of place staring at the screen of a smart phone, thus illustrating the social acceptability and validity of the technology.

Moving further into the concept of mobile technology as a self-instructional support, we should consider how many people watch videos on their mobile devices. Whether they stream a video file on YouTube or watch a movie on Netflix, they have the means to have a constant stream of information with them. Constructive use of video delivered through conventional Web sites or via purpose built software applications (apps) may permit users to have self-instructional support available to them in a wide range of environments at the point at which it is needed.

Technology can play multiple roles simultaneously to maximize outcomes for individuals with ASD. Understanding the wide range of options for how an educator or caregiver can use technology to help support an individual and subsequently help the individual support him/herself will create greater opportunities for maximizing life outcomes. However, it is important to recognize technology alone is of minimal benefit. For example, a slate and stylus were once revolutionary educational technologies, but the inert objects themselves were poor teachers. If a student was going to learn to write a sentence on the slate, a teacher had to teach him/her. If a student was going to use the slate to keep a list to help remember tasks, someone had to teach him/her. Technologies such as these are merely mediums. Teachers have to plan and arrange the environment to occasion the use of the technology and then prompt and instruct efficient use of that technology. Through this, students gain independence with the technology just as students previously gained independence with a slate and stylus. Eventually that slate and stylus evolved into notebooks, pencils, and post-it notes. In these later examples, the technology can become a prosthesis; it can provide an individual with opportunities they would not have otherwise had without the technology. As readers move through the rest of the chapter, hopefully they will note that the emphasis is not on the glitz of the technology but on the ways that the technologies are used and the means by which research shows us how to use them. The chapter will discuss mobile technology for communication and then SM more broadly.

Communication

As individuals with ASD experience difficulties with effective and appropriate social communication at varying levels (DSM-5), the use of mobile technology as an augmentative and alternative communication (AAC) device may assist individuals who have substantial support needs in communication (Chung and Douglas 2014; Shane et al. 2012; van der Meer et al. 2011). Mobile technologies now provide smaller, lighter, and cheaper AAC devices in comparison with the traditional AAC systems such as DynaVox, Tango, and GoTalk (McNaughton and Light 2013). They also have the potential to decrease the negative stigmatization often times associated with less commonplace devices which in turn could increase their adoption and usage (McNaughton and Light 2013), and decrease the potential for abandonment (Johnson et al. 2006). While there are many specialized apps to support the communication needs of individuals with ASD (Alliano et al. 2012; Bradshaw 2013; Gosnell et al. 2011), we will focus on two apps in particular—Proloquo2Go® and AutisMate.

Proloquo2Go® is a symbol-based communication app only available on Apple devices. There are over 14,000 symbols available or personalized photographs can be inserted. When a symbol or phrase is tapped, it speaks in a naturally sounding voice. The app can be easily customized to meet the vocabulary and page layout needs of individual users. Emails, texts, Tweets (via Twitter), and Facebook posts can be sent from the app also. Talk Tablet, iCommunicate, Voice4U, and iConverse are other grid-based communication apps similar to Proloquo2Go®. In the literature, elementary-age children with ASD displayed increases in reciprocal peer interactions in inclusive settings when trained to use Proloquo2Go® in conjunction with adult-mediated interaction opportunities and environmental arrangement strategies (Chung and Douglas 2014). A comparison of Proloquo2Go® on an iPad® with PECS produced mixed results (Hill and Flores 2014). The authors concluded that PECS may be the preferred communication method during early intervention and then be generalized to use on mobile devices. Additional research is needed to show the effectiveness and long-term outcomes of Proloquo2Go® and similar apps for individuals with ASD.

AutisMate is a unique app in that it promotes the development of communication and life skills. As an AAC device, it provides visual scene displays with hot spots so items can be labeled or a phrase related to the item can be spoken. Visual scene displays show images of an entire environment (e.g., a classroom) with hot spots (clickable areas) over portions of the environment that may be linked to communication. There is also a grid-based sentence builder with over 12,000 symbols that can be customized in terms of the page organization and the number and size of the symbols. This feature is similar to Proloquo2Go®. In addition to being a communication app, AutisMate provides or allows users to create video models, visual schedules with audio and videos embedded, and visual stories to support the completion of tasks at home, school, and work. AutisMate also includes a predictive keyboard and built-in GPS capabilities.

Light et al. (2004) found children aged 4–5 able to interpret meaning from both visual scene displays and grid-based displays, whereas Drager et al. (2003) and Olin et al. (2010) found younger children under three years old more successful with the visual scene over the grid screen. While these studies did not include children with ASD, the results suggest that more cognitive processing skills may be needed to interpret isolated symbols in comparison with the visual scenes with items presented in naturally occurring locations Shane (2006). Visual scenes portraying activities and events can help improve the comprehension of spoken messages as the visual picture can provide context clues (Shane 2006). Four criteria for effective visual scenes set forth by Dietz et al. (2006) include the following: (a) environmental setting, (b) interactional depiction, (c) individual relevance, and (d) clarity of scene items and their meaning. Other visual scene display apps include Scene Speak, Scene & Heard, and Touch Chat.

While AAC apps are showing great promise, we would be remiss not to mention potential challenges. First, an AAC system should be selected based on the individual's needs and skills (Beukelman and Mirenda 2013) and not because it is the latest technology fad (McNaughton and Light 2013). Second, educators and users need to learn how to operate and program the device for optimal functionality. Finally, a benefit and a challenge are devices serving multiple purposes (e.g., AAC device, visual schedule, GPS locator, and leisure games), in which the AAC app may not be able to run simultaneously with another app (King et al. 2013). This can potentially limit the accessibility and functionality of the AAC software as individuals would have to toggle between multiple apps. Even though we have to be cognizant of potential challenges, we cannot dismiss the many benefits and positive outcomes of using mobile technology with AAC apps.

Self-management

Self-management (SM) is an evidence-based practice that teaches individuals with ASD to, overtime, control their behavior (Brock 2013). Although this strategy may require an upfront investment in time and training, as the instructor fades support the learner may generalize instruction to novel environments, as well as display (similar) untrained behaviors that serve the same purpose with minimal reliance on training from staff (Lee et al. 2007). By increasing SM strategies on the job and in the community, individuals with ASD will decrease their reliance on external prompts and staff in order to follow a schedule and complete necessary tasks, thus increasing their independence (Mechling 2007).

Mechling and Savidge (2011) evaluated the use of a handheld device (i.e., PDA), in lieu of the traditional picture schedule used in the TEACCH model (Treatment and Education of Autistic and Communication Handicapped Children; Mesibov et al. 2005), as a mobile schedule for students with ASD to complete a set number of independent tasks. Students used a mobile device to view the first task, in which they could listen to an auditory prompt or watch a video model, complete the task, and then advance to the next screen to view the next task. This process was repeated until all tasks were complete, and the student was prompted (via the device) to access a preferred item. This form of mobile technology not only served as a "to-do" list, a SM tool, but it also taught the students how to complete the novel tasks (i.e., self-instruction).

Similarly, Cihak et al. (2010) taught four elementary students with ASD to navigate a handheld device (i.e., Apple video iPod®) to view video models of upcoming transitions through the school. Prior to transition, researchers provided each student with the device and instructed him or her to turn it on. Students viewed the provided video model and then lined up with their classmates. Video models of transitions presented on a handheld device increased all four students' independence with transitions while also decreasing target inappropriate behaviors (e.g., aggression, elopement, and dropping).

A traditional, hand-written to-do list does not alert you to specific times in which events must occur. For example, there are days when you must be ready (e.g., showered, dressed) by a certain time, in order to catch transportation (e.g., bus, subway, taxi), also at a specific time, to be at a set place (e.g., job, party, appointment), again at an exact time. Following this type of schedule requires the ability to respond correctly to alarms or reminders, another aspect of SM.

Davies et al. (2002) compared the efficiency of a hand-written task with a digital clock to a handheld device (i.e., Windows palmtop computer) running a scheduling program. The program provided audio and visual prompts at set times in the day. The reminders could replay automatically, upon request of the adults, or until confirmation that they completed the activity. The handheld device resulted in less assistance and fewer errors over the hand-written task list and digital clock.

In order to further increase the level of independence with the above strategy, individuals with ASD should program reminders of upcoming appointments, medication times and dosages, or other actions that need completion at set times in the day. Although specific training procedures were not provided, Gentry et al. (2010) taught high school students with ASD to input calendar entries, set reminders using the alarm function, and add contact information into the address book of a handheld device (i.e., Palm Zire 31 PDA). At the completion of the quasi-experimental study, over 80 % of the participants independently arranged prompts to self-manage.

A final component of SM in which mobile technology can replace traditional methods is in the area of self-monitoring. Self-monitoring is a strategy in which an individual changes his or her own behavior by simply becoming aware of its presence and recording the event (Maag 2004). In a general education setting, Cihak et al. (2010) trained middle school students with ASD to turn on a handheld device (i.e., HP iPAQ Mobile Media Companion handheld computer) preloaded with a PowerPoint presentation that delivered self-modeled picture prompts. Every 30 s, a picture prompt appeared on the device, showing the student engaged in target tasks (e.g., writing, reading). The student recorded on a separate note card if he or she was or was not engaged in the target behaviors. All of the students increased their task engagement, while simultaneously decreasing the number of teacher prompts required to use the device.

Self-management and self-monitoring are both considered pivotal skills in that once acquired, they increase the likelihood of collateral changes in untrained behaviors independent of additional training (Koegel et al. 1999). Some of these positive effects include generalization to novel settings, materials, and instructors, but also, and most importantly, the effects include an increase in independence and self-determined behavior. It may be a better use of instructors' and caregivers' time to focus on pivotal skills instruction. The domino effect that acquisition of a pivotal skill can have will create a much larger impact than sticking to traditional discrete trial teaching methods.

Self-instruction

Like SM, self-instruction (SI) is a pivotal skill in that once an individual has mastered a SI procedure (e.g., navigating through a phone to find a corresponding video prompt), he/she will be able to learn a variety of skills without the assistance of a caregiver or instructor (Koegel et al. 1999). For example, if an adult with ASD learns how to boil a pot of noodles using systematic instruction (e.g., least-to-most prompting), he/she will still require an instructor to then learn the remaining tasks associated with making spaghetti (e.g., how to heat up meatballs and marinara sauce). However, if an instructor successfully teaches the adult to open a video-based app on a handheld device to view videos of step-by-step directions, he or she now can complete any task in which there is a corresponding video. Thus, the adult now has the support needed to complete the chained tasks, and an instructor is not needed.

When using video models or prompts as SI tools, the planning team (e.g., learner with ASD, instructor, and others involved with program development) must consider various factors about the videos to use. The first decision involves where the video will come from. To reduce time, expertise, and efforts of support staff, a team could choose to use commercially available video from free Web sites (e.g., YouTube) or from paid packaged curricula. Although no published studies incorporate commercial videos as a SI tool (Smith et al. 2014), researchers have used commercial videos in a teacher-directed instructional arrangement to increase independence for individuals with ASD in various skill areas (Allen et al. 2010; Ayres et al. 2009). Additionally, Mechling et al. (2013) compared commercially available video prompts (i.e., "Look and Cook" software from Attainment, Inc.) to custom-made video prompts for four males with ASD using instructor-delivered video prompting. All participants reached criterion when viewing custom-made videos to cook various microwave meals, while only one participant reached 100 % correct during one session using a commercially available video. Although this is just one comparison study, these results suggest that generic and easily accessible videos may not be individualized enough for learners with ASD.

Matching specific materials, settings, and other individualized aspects of the target task are the benefits provided by custom-made videos. According to a recent review of the literature in which individuals with ID self-instructed, six studies evaluated the use of custom-made videos presented on mobile technology (Smith et al. 2014). Of the studies that used mobile technology, three included individuals with ASD learning various skills (i.e., vocational, cooking, and daily living). Mechling et al. (2009) evaluated the use of a Hewlett Packard iPAQ Pocket PC delivering picture, audio, and video prompts as a SI tool to prepare meals (i.e., Hamburger Helper, grilled ham and cheese, personal size pizza) in a school setting. Participants used a stylus or their finger to advance to a step, select prompt level(s) (i.e., picture, audio plus picture, or video), perform the step, and repeat. Also in a school setting, Bereznak et al. (2012) taught high schoolers with ASD to operate an iPhone® with video prompts to make copies, cook noodles in the microwave, and use the washing machine. Between steps in the task analyses, the iPhone® screen displayed a stop sign, signaling the participants to pause the video and complete the step. After completing each step, they pressed play on the iPhone® and repeated this pattern until task completion. Closely taking into consideration the social validity of SI, Kellems and Morningstar (2012) collaborated with adults with ASD, parents, job coaches, and employers to set target behaviors within individual job sites. Using a video iPod® set to "museum mode," participants learned to self-instruct by viewing video models prior to completing a task at work. Participants placed earbuds in so as not to disturb customers and coworkers, turned on the iPod®, and selected the corresponding video to the target task.

Although the creation of custom videos does not have to take a lot of time, some caregivers and instructors still report hesitation in that they do not want to create a separate video for each task an individual needs to learn (Rosenberg et al. 2010). In addition to the reluctance to create videos, relying on support staff to create custom videos somewhat defeats the goal of SI. In order to fully eliminate reliance on others, individuals with ASD must learn to create their own instructional materials needed to self-instruct. Each day people create their own SI materials to complete individual tasks (e.g., write down recipes, print out driving directions) and series of tasks (e.g., write down to-do list, input meetings and dates into electronic calendars). Duttlinger et al. (2012) used least-to-most promoting to teach four middle school students, one with ASD, to create their own picture to-do list. As the teacher explained three to five tasks that needed completion, students placed corresponding BoardMaker pictures onto a strip of paper affixed with Velcro. The researchers used a withdrawal design to evaluate the use of the picture schedule, demonstrating an increased percentage of correct responses (i.e., placing the correct picture on the list and completing tasks in the correct order) when the picture to-do list was in place compared to just using short-term memory to follow through with all tasks (i.e., no picture schedule). Expanding on this research while moving forward with current technology, Uphold et al. (2014) used constant time delay (CTD) to teach six adults (two with ASD) to program a picture-based first-then workout schedule using an iPod® Touch. Adults participating in the study first took pictures of their peers engaging in 14 different exercises (e.g., walk 2 laps, 10 push ups) to build a bank of photographs. Once the instructor started to state the exercises required for the day, they were to turn on the mobile technology, locate the first-then app, and add exercise pictures in the order stated by the instructor. All participants reached criterion in programing the iPod® and all increased levels of correct exercise responding when they used the electronic picture schedule (i.e., user created prompt with mobile technology).

Shepley et al. (2014) examined the use of video modeling to teach four high school students (two with ASD) to record their own videos using an iPhone®. Prior to each intervention session, participants viewed a video model of an actor going through the necessary steps to access the camera app on an iPhone® and record a video. Three of the four students acquired the skill of creating their own self-prompting materials (i.e., a video model) and generalized it to a novel setting. At the completion of the study, a quick social validity measure was conducted in which students independently filmed a video of the researcher performing a novel skill (i.e., using a laminator). Students acquired at least 50 % of steps after viewing their self-made video one time. Further experimental validations are required to evaluate the acquisition of novel tasks using student-created prompts; however, the field is heading in the right direction to further increase independence in individuals with ASD and fade instructor support.

Challenges

Now that the field of special education recognizes the importance and value of SM and SI for individuals with ASD, the next question then becomes, "How do we teach children, adolescents, or adults with ASD to use the technology?" Simply handing over the technology, whether it is novel or not, does not mean a learner will use it resourcefully, or that they will even use it at all. Just like when learning any new skill, teachers and caregivers must use systematic instruction to teach the proper use of the technology.

Although not specific to SI, Hammond et al. (2010) taught three middle students with ID to watch a movie, listen to music, and look at photographs using a third-generation iPod® Nano. This study demonstrated that with systematic instruction (i.e., video modeling), young children with ID could navigate mobile technology. When the video modeling prompt was removed, correct responding was not maintained; however, booster sessions brought responding backup to criterion levels. To further expand the use of video modeling to increase mobile technology navigation, Walser et al. (2012) taught high school students with ID to watch a video, look at pictures, and take a picture with an iPhone® 3GS. Additional prompts (i.e., "Don't hold so long") were provided to one participant who touched the icons for an extended duration, which caused the phone to go into edit mode. Another participant was hesitant to touch the mobile device, in fear of breaking it; therefore, a researcher demonstrated how strong and durable the device was when in its protective case.

In the Smith et al. (2014) review of SI, the majority of studies (i.e., 42 %) used history training to expose the individuals with ID to the SI technologies prior to the study starting. Various forms of systematic instruction (i.e., least-to-most prompting, verbal plus model prompting, and model prompting alone) were implemented with a task not targeted for SI. Participants completed history training once they responded at criterion levels, such as three sessions at 100 % correct responding. Although this is common practice when introducing an individual to a novel independent variable, a lack of reported data on this process is a huge limitation in the existing research. Without this data, we cannot recommend the most efficient systematic instruction, including types of prompts and how often to prompt when teaching an individual with ID or ASD to self-instruct.

Another gap in the existing literature pertains to teaching individuals with ASD to identify the need to use the support. This includes acknowledging that assistance is needed (e.g., a video prompt from a handheld device), as well as initiating the use of a prompting system (e.g., pulling the device out of your pocket and locating the video). Currently, published studies that used some form of SI included information about the prompting system in the discriminative stimulus (Smith et al. 2014). For example, when given the task demand to "stock the vending machine," participants were either provided an additional verbal prompt (e.g., to "use your phone,") or were handed the device following the task direction. In both of these examples, the participant did not have to identify the need to use the device or initiate the use.

Smith (2014) systematically faded additional instructor prompts to increase independent initiations to use SI technology and programmed for generalization across environments and instructors for high school students with ASD. During history training, students were taught to navigate an iPhone® to locate video prompts. Prior to all sessions, participants placed an iPhone® in their pocket so it was in their possession during probes. The start of each probe began with a task direction (e.g., set up the board game, pierce the potato), and the dependent measures included initiating retrieving and navigating the device, as well as percentage correct of task completion. After delivering the task demand, the instructor used progressive time delay (i.e., PTD, 0–3 s) to deliver the controlling prompt (i.e., "Get your phone our and watch a video about —"). Participants required instruction (i.e., PTD) to initiate and self-instruct in an initial environment (e.g., kitchen, office, or courtyard), and later generalized these skills across multiple environments and instructors (i.e., classroom teacher). Smith and colleagues successfully removed the adult prompt to self-instruct from the discriminative stimulus. Also, by programming for generalization, the participants in this study had the opportunity to learn a large variety of skills across environments with SI alone.

One additional challenge is the accessibility of mobile technology for persons with ASD. Possible upfront activations costs and monthly payments to service providers may inhibit use by some individuals; therefore, the cost-benefit ratio may need to be considered. Along with the cost, the fear of damaging a device can be a barrier for individuals with ASD or persons purchasing the device (e.g., caregivers, school systems). While breaking a device is possible for anyone using mobile technology, teaching skills related to responsibility and care for belongings provides opportunities for learning additional independent living skills.

Technology on the Horizon

Technology is changing on a daily basis. As technology advances, it is becoming more readily available and accessible for individuals with ASD. These technologies have the potential to continually improve the independence and quality of life for people with ASD and other disabilities. Examples of technology on the horizon include geo-location systems, radio frequency (RF) tags, and augmented reality. These are discussed below as their applicability and usefulness for individuals with ASD and their families continue to grow.

Geo-location-based supports allow you to find and track the location of your child inside and outside the home. Alerts in the form of a flashing light, alarm, or vibration will let you know when your child has approached the maximum distance you programmed into the device such as a road, pool, or perimeter of a store (called geo-fencing) or allow you to find them in a crowded room. Some systems provide two-way voice communication. A few examples of these tracking systems include iCare, Trax, Amber Alert GPS, and Spark Nano 4.0. Each system should be further researched as they all have different capabilities and costs.

RF tags are enabling PECS users to bring sound to the symbols through the use of a Logan® ProxTalker® communication device. This device has RF identification technology that reads sound tags on vocabulary symbols to produce the spoken word. While PECS is an effective AAC system, this device allows individuals to communicate even when their communication partner is not looking at them or is not close enough to make a picture exchange.

Finally, augmented reality is changing how people access information in their daily lives and at school. By orienting a mobile phone toward the sky, a user can identify and learn about the stars and constellations using apps such as Google Sky Map, Starlight, or Star Chart. As another example, a learner can point the camera of a mobile device over a flashcard, and AR Flashcards (www.arflashcards.com) provide sound and images to increase the salience and interest level of conventional materials. Ultimately, augmented reality overlays an image with digital information viewed on a device. It enables individuals to play basketball (AR Basketball) or soccer (AR Soccer) on their mobile device in their free time. Augmented Car Finder shows where your car is parked. In addition, Trax, a GPS tracking system, also includes an augmented reality feature through the use of your device's camera. You turn in a circle until you see a logo on the camera screen that represents the direction of the tracker and tells you the distance between you and it. This feature can help you locate a child without having to read a map.

Conclusions

Technology evolution has given us greater flexibility and opportunity. Learning to navigate by stars allowed sailors to traverse great distances just as the development of the compass created greater opportunity for people to engage with other cultures as they traveled beyond their own countries. When technology becomes mobile, it begs us to join our community and it can free us from the safety of home. As you have read in this chapter, technology can be a powerful teaching tool. It can also be a very useful companion when one is trying to achieve greater independence in the community. Mobile phones replaced pay phones and are now beginning to replace GPSs. We no longer have to search for a quarter and maps are becoming quaint relics. We have a wealth of information literally in the palms of our hands.

The pervasiveness of mobile technology means that no one stands out from the crowd if they are using a mobile device (phone or tablet). Further, as individuals with ASD come to represent an important part of this market share, innovation will follow. Technologies designed to serve the needs of an individual with ASD (e.g., communication, SM, or SI) can benefit a wider audience. The versatility and flexibility of having a powerful computer in your pocket creates opportunities. To take advantage of those opportunities, however, individuals need to learn to use the technology and they need to have access to the technology. While cost and accessibility will always be an obstacle, educators can employ evidence-based practices to ensure that they are teaching end users in the most appropriate manner.

References

Allen, K. D., Wallace, D. P., & Renes, D. (2010). Use of video modeling to teach vocational skills to adolescents and young adults with autism spectrum disorders. *Education and Treatment of Children, 33*, 339–349.

Alliano, A., Herriger, K., Koutsoftas, A. D., & Bartolotta, T. E. (2012). A review of 21 iPad applications for augmentative and alternative communication purposes. *Perspectives on Augmentative and Alternative Communication, 21*(2), 60–71.

American Heritage Dictionary (4th ed.). (2000). Boston: Houghlin Mifflin Company.

Ayres, K. M., Maguire, A., & McClimon, D. (2009). Acquisition and generalization of chained tasks taught with computer based video instruction to children with autism. *Education and Training in Developmental Disabilities, 44*, 493–508.

Ayres, K. M., Shepley, C., & Douglas, K. H. (2014, in press). Assistive and instructional technology for individuals with autism. In. R. Simpson (Ed.). *Educating Children and Youth with Autism: Strategies for Effective Practice.*

Bereznak, S., Ayres, K. M., Mechling, L. C., & Alexander, J. L. (2012). Video self-prompting and mobile technology to increase daily living and vocational independence for students with autism spectrum disorders. *Journal of Developmental and Physical Disabilities, 24*, 269–285.

Beukelman, D., & Mirenda, P. (2013). *Augmentative and alternative communication: Supporting children and adults with complex communication needs* (4th ed.). Baltimore, MD: Paul Brookes Publishing Co.

Bradshaw, J. (2013). The use of augmentative and alternative communication apps for the iPad, iPod and iPhone: An overview of recent developments. *Tizard Learning Disability Review, 18*, 31–37.

Brock, M. E. (2013). *Self-management (SM) fact sheet.* Chapel Hill: The University of North Carolina, Frank Porter Graham Child Development Institute, The National Professional Development Center on Autism Spectrum Disorders.

Chung, Y. C. & Douglas, K. H. (2014, in review). Paraprofessional-delivered strategies to increase interactions of students who use Proloquo2go in inclusive classrooms.

Cihak, D., Fahrenkroq, C., Ayres, K. M., & Smith, C. (2010a). The use of video modeling via a video iPod and a system of least prompts to improve transitional behaviors for students with autism spectrum disorders in the general education setting. *Journal of Positive Behavior Interventions, 12*, 103–115.

Cihak, D. F., Wright, R., & Ayres, K. M. (2010b). Use of self-modeling static-picture prompts via a handheld computer to facilitate self-monitoring in the general education classroom. *Education and Training in Autism and Developmental Disabilities, 45*, 136–149.

Davies, D. K., Stock, S. E., & Wehmeyer, M. L. (2002). Enhancing independent time-management skills on individuals with mental retardation using a palm-op personal computer. *Mental Retardation, 40*, 358–365.

Dietz, A., McKelvey, M., Hux, K., Beukelman, D., Wallace, S., & Weissling, K. (2006, November). *Integrating contextual relevant visual scenes into aphasia interventions.* Paper presented at the Annual Convention of the American Speech-Language-Hearing Association, Miami Beach, FL.

Drager, K. D. R., Light, J. C., Curran Speltz, J., Fallon, K. A., & Jeffries, L. Z. (2003). The performance of typically developing 2 ½-year-olds on dynamic display AAC technologies with different system layouts and language organizations. *Journal of Speech Language Hearing Research, 46*, 298–312.

Duttlinger, C., Ayres, K. M., Bevill-Davis, A., & Douglas, K. H. (2012). The effects of a picture activity schedule for students with intellectual disability to complete a sequence of tasks following verbal directions. *Focus on Autism and Other Developmental Disabilities, 28*, 32–43.

Gentry, T., Wallace, J., Kvarfordt, C., & Lynch, K. B. (2010). Personal digital assistants as cognitive aids for high school students with autism: Results of a community-based trial. *Journal of Vocational Rehabilitation, 32*, 101–107.

Gosnell, J., Costello, J., & Shane, H. (2011). There isn't always an app for that! *Perspectives on Augmentative and Alternative Communication, 20*, 7–8. doi:10.1044/aac20.1.7.

Hammond, D. L., Whatley, A. D., Ayres, K. M., & Gast, D. L. (2010). Effectiveness of video modeling to teach iPod use to students with moderate intellectual disabilities. *Education and Training in Developmental Disabilities, 45*, 525–538.

Hill, D. A., & Flores, M. M. (2014). Comparing the picture exchange communication system and the iPad for communication of students with autism spectrum disorder and developmental delay. *TechTrends, 58*(3), 45–53.

Johnson, J. M., Inglebret, E., Jones, C., & Ray, J. (2006). Perspectives of speech language pathologists regarding success versus abandonment of AAC. *Augmentative and Alternative Communication, 22*, 85–99.

Kellems, R. O., & Morningstar, M. E. (2012). Video modeling using iPods to teach vocational tasks to young adults with autism spectrum disorders. *Career Development and Transition for Exceptional Individuals, 35*, 155–167.

King, A. M., Thomeczek, M., Voreis, G., & Scott, V. (2013). iPad use in children and young adults with autism spectrum disorder: An observational study. *Child Language Teaching and Therapy, 30*, 159–173. doi:10.1177/0265659013510922.

Koegel, L. K., Koegel, R. L., Harrower, J. K., & Carter, C. M. (1999). Pivotal response intervention I: Overview of approach. *Journal of the Association of Persons with Severe Handicaps, 24*, 174–185.

Lee, S. H., Simpson, R. L., & Shogren, K. A. (2007). Effects and implications of self-management for students with autism: A meta-analysis. *Focus on Autism and Other Developmental Disabilities, 22*, 2–13.

Light, J., Drager, K., McCarthy, J., Mellott, S., Parrish, C., Parsons, A., et al. (2004). Performance of typically developing four and five year old children with AAC systems using different language organization techniques. *Augmentative and Alternative Communication, 20*, 63–88.

Linsley, O. R. (1964). Direct measurement and prosthesis of retarded behavior. *Journal of Education, 147*, 62–81.

Maag, J. W. (2004). *Behavior management: From theoretical implication to practical applications* (2nd ed.). Belmont, CA: Wadsworth/Thomas Learning.

McNaughton, D., & Light, J. (2013). The iPad and mobile technology revolution: Benefits and challenges for individuals who require augmentative and alternative communication. *Augmentative and Alternative Communication, 29*, 107–116.

Mechling, L. C. (2007). Assistive technology as a self-management tool for prompting students with intellectual disabilities to initiate and complete daily tasks: A literature review. *Education and Training in Developmental Disabilities, 42*, 252–269.

Mechling, L. C., & Savidge, E. J. (2011). Using a personal digital assistant to increase completion of novel tasks and independent transitioning by students with autism spectrum disorder. *Journal on Autism and Developmental Disorders, 41*, 687–704.

Mechling, L. C., & Stephens, E. (2009). Comparison of self-prompting of cooking skills via picture-based cookbooks and video recipes. *Education and Training in Developmental Disabilities, 44*, 218–236.

Mechling, L. C., Gast, D. L., & Seid, N. H. (2009). Using a personal digital assistant to increase independent task completion by students with autism spectrum disorder. *Journal of Autism and Developmental Disorders, 39*, 1420–1434.

Mechling, L. C., Ayres, K. M., Foster, A. L., & Bryant, K. J. (2013). Comparing the effects of commercially available and custom-made video prompting for teaching cooking skills to high school students with autism. *Remedial and Special Education, 34*, 371–383.

Mesibov, G. B., Shea, V., & Schopler, E. (2005). *The TEACCH approach to autism spectrum disorders*. New York, NY: Kluwer Academic/Plenum Publishers.

Olin, A. R., Reichle, J., Johnson, L., & Monn, E. (2010). Examining dynamic visual scene displays: Implications for arranging and teaching symbol selection. *American Journal of Speech-Language Pathology, 19*, 284–297.

Rosenberg, N. E., Schwartz, I. S., & Davis, C. A. (2010). Evaluating the utility of commercial videotapes for teaching hand washing to children with autism. *Education and Treatment of Children, 33*, 443–455.

Shane, H. C. (2006). Using visual scene displays to improve communication and communication instruction in persons with autism spectrum disorders. *Perspectives on Augmentative and Alternative Communication, 15*, 7–13.

Shane, H., Laubscher, E., Schlosser, R., Flynn, S., Sorce, J., & Abramson, J. (2012). Applying technology to visually support language and communication in individuals with autism spectrum disorders. *Journal of Autism and Developmental Disorders, 42*, 1228–1235. doi:10.1007/s10803-011-1304-z.

Shepley, S. B., Smith, K. A., Ayres, K. M., & Alexander, J. L. (2014, unpublished manuscript). The use of video modeling to teach adolescents with intellectual disability to film their own video prompts.

Smith, K. A. (2014). *Initiation and generalization of self-instructional skills.* (Unpublished doctoral dissertation). The University of Georgia, Athens.

Taber-Doughty, T. (2005). Considering student choice when selecting instructional strategies: A comparison of three prompting systems. *Research in Developmental Disabilities, 26*, 411–432.

Uphold, N. M., Douglas, K. H., & Loseke, D. L. (2014, in press). Effects of using an iPod app to manage recreation tasks. *Career Development and Transition for Exceptional Individuals.*

van der Meer, L., Kagohara, D., Achmadi, D., Green, V. A., Herrington, C., Sigafoos, J., et al. (2011). Teaching functional use of an iPod-based speech-generating device to students with developmental disabilities. *Journal of Special Education Technology, 26*(3), 1–11.

Walser, K., Ayres, K., & Foote, E. (2012). Effects of a video model to teach students with moderate intellectual disability to use key features of an iPhone. *Education and Training in Autism and Developmental Disabilities, 47*, 319–331.

Wolery, M., & Hemmeter, M. L. (2011). Classroom instruction: Background, assumptions, and challenges. *Journal of Early Intervention, 33*, 371–380. doi:10.1177/1053815111429119.

Chapter 12
An Insider's Look at Technology and Autism

Tricia Nelson and Riley's Mom

As a baby, Riley grew and developed right on track. He seemed to hit all of his milestones like a champ. There was one thing that we noticed that seemed different from other toddlers his age… his early development of speech. He babbled early on. He began saying "mamma" and "dadda" at around 8 months. At 11 months, he would say "t-anks" (thanks) when given something that he wanted, and his language continued to progress from there. At 12 months of age, he began walking and his talking increased. His pronunciation was incredible. Hearing him say words such as "Elmo" and "milk" when he was so tiny was fun for us. By 16 months, he could sing the alphabet, say all the animal sounds, count to 5 and much more.

But around 18 months of age, his language took a steep decline. By 23 months, he had only a few words in his vocabulary and he was officially diagnosed with autism. It was devastating for our family. However, we decided that it was time to get to work trying to recover as much of our Riley-man as we could.

Our first encounter with speech therapy was our journey through the Picture Exchange Communication System (PECS). In the beginning, it seemed to work well. After a short time, he could find his picture and bring it to us. The struggle came with discriminating between preferred and non-preferred items. We presented items including a piece of candy and a piece of broccoli. Riley would reach for the picture of broccoli, and when handed the piece of broccoli, he would simply play with it and let it entertain him. It was clear he wanted the candy, but it did not upset him not to get it. Even when working with his "most preferred" items, he just did not seem to care much about which card he handed us and what the result was of his communication. Another roadblock we hit was trying to find pictures of each of the things he could request, therefore giving him options. We ended up with hundreds of cards and a binder full of options, with no real functional way to use them. Add to that, carrying around the binder with all of the pictures, and PECS, just did not pan out as a functional communication option for Riley.

For years after a very diligent struggle with PECS, we decided to put an even stronger emphasis on verbal language and sign language. Riley was taught basic

T. Nelson (✉) · R. Mom
Utah Autism Academy, Midvale, UT, USA
e-mail: tnelson@utahautismacademy.com

© Springer International Publishing Switzerland 2016
T.A. Cardon (ed.), *Technology and the Treatment of Children with Autism Spectrum Disorder*, Autism and Child Psychopathology Series, DOI 10.1007/978-3-319-20872-5_12

147

sign and could imitate almost any sign we used. However, his ability to use it independently was hampered by his poor receptive language skills. He would match the verbal cue of "cookie" with the appropriate sign, but would really want a drink. If we said "drink," he would sign it (without a visual prompt), even if we had a cookie in front of him as the desired item. Needless to say, his nonverbal imitation skills got really good, but his ability to use sign language for meeting his needs just did not fit.

By the time he was about 10 years of age, we decided that a financial investment in an iPad (although money was tight) was necessary. Little did we know that it would be worth its weight in gold. Riley's ability to navigate through the programs on the iPad was incredible! One of the first apps that his behavioral therapist downloaded was a learning app called "See, Touch, Learn." With this app, we were able to create our own games (with our own images and voice prompts), create custom lessons, and give opportunities for Riley to navigate around thousands of pictures, giving us an insight into his interests. He really enjoyed it.

By about the age of 11, Riley was given options on his iPad for communication. The app that we used was "Quick Talk." We started simple, with just a few pictures. He picked up on it, slowly but surely. As his understanding of the concept grew, we began to add an array of pictures of Disney movies. He loved looking at it. Then, he would scroll them and touch one of his favorites. We would immediately turn on the movie that he had requested. He was thrilled. He started using it to communicate his wants for movies more often. Handing him an iPad and prompting him to choose what he wanted would stop a meltdown in its tracks! Although his communication on his device was limited, it would continue to grow.

Now, at the age of 13, Riley uses his iPad on a regular basis to get basic wants met. We have switched to a program called "Bitsboard" as it is being widely used with other students in his therapy program. Although, he is not able to completely express his needs and desires yet, it is clear that it makes him feel empowered to be able to share basic wants through his limited use of the iPad.

One thought that has stuck out to me through this process is that I was convinced that if we had him use his iPad for communication, rather than pushing vocalizations, we had accepted to the fact that he would never talk. My thoughts could not have been further from the truth. Since he has increased his use of the iPad, his vocalizations have increased like I would not have imagined. He is not saying full sentences, but for the first time in years, we are hearing words! One word that he says, almost clearer than any other, is "iPad." Becoming familiar with the deep voice of our 13-year-old son is something I had dreams about before… but, now is a reality.

Since the iPad has become a constant companion for Riley, we have also had the opportunity to try new things with it. Using his iPad for tracking of his programs has been very helpful as well. In Riley's "Day Treatment" program, they use an iPad app known as "Catalyst." The staff are able to pull up specific programs, note current goals and prompt history as well as refer to any modifications or notes on specific targets. Not only does this program hold all of his treatment plan information, it also includes personal information, home notes, and so much more.

The therapists carry the iPad around all day and are able to access all of his programs and record data that can be viewed real time by supervisory staff and parents. The capabilities it has to graph the information with just a click of a button allow for opportunities to analyze behaviors and see marked growth or difficulty without spending hours compiling written data for charting. The staff also use this iPad to video record many of his programs so that I can see his progress and share it with others. One of my favorites is when video clips are sent to me that include Riley speaking.

Riley also enjoys participating in video-modeling sessions and enjoys using it in "selfie mode" for emotions and nonverbal facial imitation programs. Having the immediate access to an iPad for video modeling has been not only productive for Riley's learning and growth, but also for his entertainment! He loves to learn through watching others and himself. Many times, his therapists, peers and even siblings will video themselves singing his favorite Disney songs. This has proven to be a great way for him to practice his verbal imitation skills. It is fun to watch he and a staff member in "selfie mode" singing "You've got a friend in me"! Recording it is fun... watching it play back is even more fun.

For some of Riley's fine motor programs, they use a program called "Letter School." Although it is not a complicated program or fancy app, Riley (and so many others) is drawn to this program. The immediate prompt fading techniques that the app uses for more immediate independence of skills seem to work for him. When given spare time on his iPad, this is certainly an app that he is drawn to.

His iPad has been used for reinforcement as well. He loves watching Disney clips! Also, there is a YouTube channel where an adult female records herself opening chocolate Kinder eggs that have a surprise inside. Riley gets so excited and can hardly contain his anticipation! This is specifically helpful because chocolate Kinder eggs are not available for sale in the USA. So, being able to access the videos on his iPad is extremely helpful and highly motivating for Riley. I was also surprised to hear that several of the kids in his program are drawn to the same YouTube channel!

Overall, the use of technology for Riley's growth and development has played a monumental role. I cannot imagine living without it. As technology changes, we continue to explore options for learning and communication apps that will help him progress to a place of better functionality in society.

Chapter 13
A Look Forward

Teresa A. Cardon

The speed at which technology is changing and advancing continues at an unprecedented rate. At the time of this writing, the annual Consumer Electronics Show (CES) in Las Vegas just ended (January 2015). Advances in technology ranged from clothing equipped with Bluetooth devices to smart refrigerators to 4K televisions. Given the rate at which technology is changing, it is difficult to predict the future of technology and autism. It is possible to predict, however, that the promising path of technological support for individuals with ASD will continue to alter their lives in ways we may not even have imagined yet. In addition to the future technological possibilities mentioned in Chap. 11, this final chapter will briefly touch on innovations that are starting to cross paths with autism.

Apps

While apps are not new to autism, the plethora of apps that provide intervention and support for children with ASD will continue to grow and advance. Recently, Samsung announced the new "Look at Me" app that is designed to help children with autism improve the "ability to make eye contact" (http://pages.samsung.com/ca/lookatme/English/). The app was developed by a team of psychologists and psychiatrists and is currently undergoing clinical testing. In addition, families that are using the app are connected through the Look at Me Project (2015), a shared community similar to a social media experiment, where families can share the progress their children are making.

A soon to be released app, developed with the help of MIT's Media Lab, focuses on emotion reading software that will help children with ASD identify emotions. Affectiva (www.affectiva.com) software analyzes images of faces and can detect nuances such as furrowed brows and smirks. Children with ASD will be able to submit pictures of faces in order to get a description of the mood depicted in the picture. The software database

T.A. Cardon (✉)
Utah Valley University, Orem, UT, USA
e-mail: Teresa.cardon@uvu.edu

© Springer International Publishing Switzerland 2016
T.A. Cardon (ed.), *Technology and the Treatment of Children with Autism Spectrum Disorder*, Autism and Child Psychopathology Series,
DOI 10.1007/978-3-319-20872-5_13

currently holds more than a billion facial expressions and will provide support to children with ASD as they learn to analyze and understand emotions.

Wearables

Google Glass became available to the public in May of 2014. Since that time, the number of companies testing and developing software for the wearable product has quickly expanded. There are several intriguing elements of Google Glass that can offer support for individuals with ASD. One aspect that has particular promise is the real-time aspect of interactions that can be supported with Google Glass. For example, there are several software programs that can help individuals with autism identify facial expressions and emotions. Natasha Jaques, a PhD student at the Massachusetts Institute of Technology Media Lab, is studying how to support social interactions between people with autism by providing social cues based on facial expressions. For example, if someone appears bored with a conversation, the software would alert the user wearing Google Glass that the listener is becoming bored (Melynchuck 2015).

Ned Sahin, a scientist and the CEP of Brain Power, is in the process of testing a variety of Google Glass apps to support learning in children with ASD. He believes that the future of wearable technology will unlock social interactions for children with autism (Autism Speaks 2014). Brain Power is researching how to support increased eye contact, how to teach emotion recognition, and how to match a facial expression to an emotion all with the use of Google Glass.

Another wearable technology that is still considered brand new at the time of this writing is a smart watch. Most smart watches sync with a smartphone and provide the user with apps and access to instant messaging. It has been hypothesized that smart watches will be able to provide the type of structure that can support increased executive functioning skills in individuals with ASD. Reminders and visual schedules will appear on someone's wrist to help direct them throughout their day. For added benefit, smart watch vibrations will accompany reminders to increase awareness of appointments, important things that should not be forgotten like medication, etc. This type of increased support can decrease anxiety and increase communication opportunities for individuals with ASD.

In addition, smart watches and other wearable devices are integral safety elements that are currently being expanded to address elopement issues for children with ASD. Wearables with global positioning technology can offer peace of mind for parents if they have a child with ASD who tends to wander off. While there are several different types of wearable trackers (Revolutionary Tracker, EZ100 Personal Emergency Notifier, Independence Day Clothing, etc.), they all serve a similar purpose in providing direct location information for the child with ASD. Some devices even allow a parent to set a predetermined distance that, when breached, will trigger the wearable device to vibrate and an alert on the parents smartphone to notify them that a child has travelled too far away (Autism Speaks 2015).

Similar to a smart watch, research is currently being conducted on wearable sensor technology to track "autism in action" (Yandell 2015). Similar to fitness trackers that track heart rate and steps, wearable sensors may be able to predict when a child is getting agitated by tracking heart rate, movement, sleep, and sweat levels. The idea is that by monitoring a child's actions on a daily basis, physiological information will provide insights into when a child may be overwhelmed or getting frustrated. The ultimate goal of wearable sensors would be to predict when dangerous or disruptive behaviors are about to occur so that parents and clinicians can intervene beforehand to keep individuals with autism safe.

Robots

Future technological advances for children with ASD will also include robots.

It is believed that robots may be able to support social development in children with ASD because the uncertainty and sense of being overwhelmed that can accompany live interactions is limited, allowing a child to focus on targeted social cues and directions. For example, Milo is a two-foot-tall robot that is the innovation of a former Disney imagineer, David Hanson. Milo can be programmed with a script that is predetermined for an interaction with a child, or Milo can be controlled by an operator or a therapist to interact spontaneously with a child with ASD (Tucker 2015). Milo's eyes record a child's facial expressions and eye contact, while other monitors on the child capture their heart rate to determine varying levels of stress involved during the interaction. Interactions with robots to support learning and skill development in children with ASD may be more effective and less stress inducing than interactions with similarly aged peers (Edmiston et al. 2014). The future of robot technology may allow for children with ASD to learn target skills while interacting with a robot before going on to generalize those skills with a peer.

It is impossible to predict how technological advances over the next 20 years will change and alter the lives of individuals with ASD; however, if future technology develops anywhere near as fast and uniquely as it has in the past 20 years, the possibilities seem truly limitless.

References

Autism Speaks. (2014). *Scientist to begin beta testing Google glass autism apps next year.* Retrieved February 15, 2015, from http://www.autismspeaks.org/news/news-item/scientist-begin-beta-testing-google-glass-autism-apps-next-year.

Autism Speaks. (2015). *Safety products.* Retrieved February 15, 2015, from http://www.autismspeaks.org/family-services/resource-library/safety-products.

Edmiston, E. K., Merkle, K., & Corbett, B. A. (2014). Neural and cortisol responses during play with human and computer partners in children with autism. *Social cognitive and affective neuroscience*, 159.

Melynchuck, M. (2015). *U of R grad's studies utilize Google Glass.* Leader Post retrieved February 15, 2015, from http://www.leaderpost.com/health/grad+studies+utilize+Google +Glass+Video/10701648/story.html#__federated=1.

The Look at Me Project. (2015). Retrieved January 20, 2015, from http://pages.samsung.com/ca/lookatme/English/.

Tucker, E. (2015). *How robots are helping children with autism. The Guardian.* Retrieved February 2, 2015, from http://www.theguardian.com/lifeandstyle/2015/feb/01/how-robots-helping-children-with-autism.

Yandell, K. (2015). *Wearable sensors aim to capture autism in action.* Retrieved February 20, 2015, from http://sfari.org/news-and-opinion/blog/2015/wearable-sensors-aim-to-capture-autism-in-action.

Index

Note: Page numbers followed by "f" and "t" indicate figures and tables respectively

Printed in Great Britain
by Amazon